ENERGY EATING:
The Vegetarian Way

Lucy Moll

A Perigee Book

Most Perigee Books are available at special quantity discounts for bulk
purchases for sales promotions, premiums, fund-raising, or educational use.
Special books or book excerpts can also be created to fit specific needs.

For details, write to: Special Markets, The Berkley Publishing Group, 375
Hudson Street, New York, New York 10014.

A Perigee Book
Published by The Berkley Publishing Group
A division of Penguin Putnam Inc.
375 Hudson Street,
New York, New York 10014

Copyright © 1999 by Lucy Moll
Book design by Lisa Stokes
Cover design by Miguel Santana
Cover photograph copyright © by The Stock Market/Walter Swarthout

First edition: July 1999

Published simultaneously in Canada.

The Penguin Putnam Inc. World Wide Web site address is
http://www.penguinputnam.com

Library of Congress Cataloging-in-Publication Data
Moll, Lucy.
Energy eating : the vegetarian way / Lucy Moll. — 1st ed.
p.   cm.
"A Perigee book."
ISBN 0-399-52512-2
1. Vegetarianism.   2. Functional foods.   3. Nutrition.   4. Health.
I. Title.
RM236.M65   1999
613.2'62—dc21   98-56394
                                                           CIP

Printed in the United States of America

10 9 8 7 6 5 4 3 2 1

For Julia, my forever child,
a gift of the Gift-Giver
whose greatest power
is the Word

acknowledgments

This book would not be in your hands but for my personal "assistants" who graced me in amazing ways.

Steve, Laura and Julia . . . Wow! Your love overwhelms me. I couldn't have done this without you.

Rob and Becky Fletcher, Tim and Jan Miller, and Pam and Mike Zeidman . . . Our friendship has made me a better person and writer, for through you I have experienced truth. An *authentic* thanks!

Steve Persson . . . You've been an inspiration. If you thought the Afterword struck a chord, just wait 'til my next book. It'll sing.

Jim Cofield . . . I greatly appreciate your feedback on several chapters but, more important, I thank you for your presence and passion.

Derek Chignell . . . Your review of this book, and especially your comments on the biochemistry sections, were indispensable to its improvement. Any and all mistakes, confusions and incomplete or misleading information are solely my own.

Katy Kang . . . What could I possibly say that would capture my sisterly love for you? Thanks for your review of these chapters and for your wisdom and encouragement.

I also extend my gratitude to Ted Piton, Mary Moll, Carolyn Winter, Jennifer Ochs, Rema D'Alessandro, John and Maria Shalanko, Wes and Beth Wetherall, Lora Helton, Beth Larson, and the editors (past and present) of *Vegetarian Times* magazine—as well as to my agent, Angela Miller, and editor, Dolores Mc-Mullan—all of whom made valuable contributions.

Finally, to my Lord and Savior, I pray that all who hear your voice will open the doors of their hearts so you will be exalted, for without you we are lost and with you, well, that's another story.

contents

What's in a Promise?

We make promises all the time.

"I'll take out the trash."

"I'll have the report on your desk by noon."

"I'll scrub the bathtub grout."

"I'll love you until death do us part."

Yet we break them often: We choose *Seinfeld* reruns over throwing out the garbage or beautifying the lavatory. We finish the report late. We divorce.

A promise is simply a declaration of what one will do or refrain from doing.

To this end, *Energy Eating* has an underlying give-and-take message. It *gives* a promise to unlock a door for you, the door that opens to a powered-up mind, mood, and body via three pathways—power-eating, power-cise, and power-living—with the greatest emphasis on food, delicious food. This book won't solve all of life's problems, mind you. But it'll put you in a healthier place to face them.

It asks you to *take* up the promise, to embrace it. In accepting it fully, you make an unspoken promise in return: to choose to care for yourself.

Give and take. My responsibility, your responsibility. That is what it comes down to, really.

This book came together with the blending of my interests

in researching the brain, particularly neurotransmitters, the bio-chemical messengers that pass vital chunks of information among brain cells, and in developing vegetarian recipes. It sounds like a strange mix, doesn't it?

But the more I researched and the more I cooked and the more I ate, I observed that some foods lifted my mood while others seemed to make me lethargic or uptight. One day stands out in particular.

On the morning I was scheduled to appear on a television interview show as an expert on the vegetarian diet, I woke up with the jitters. My mind did the "monkey," with thoughts jumping frenetically from tree limb to tree limb inside my skull. My mood went along for the wild ride into anxiety.

By this point in my research, I knew of the work of Richard and Judith Wurtman, a husband-wife team at the Massachusetts Institute of Technology. They were the first to look at how food affects neurotransmitters and, in turn, mood. In my frenzied state, I somehow managed to ask myself, "What would the Wurtmans suggest I eat for breakfast to calm my mood and mind?" The answer: carbohydrates, eaten without any high-protein food.

Luckily, I had a chocolate-chip bagel stashed in my freezer. I warmed it and enjoyed it without guilt, for chocolate is suspected to trigger the feel-good endorphins. By the time I reached the TV studio in downtown Chicago, I felt at ease and not at all nervous.

As these chapters unfold, you'll see why the latest research into the highly complex, still-mysterious brain points to this most amazing discovery: Eating the right foods at the right times in the right combinations can help you think, feel, and physically perform your very best, whenever you choose.

The "right" foods aren't esoteric, weird, or terribly expensive. They're vegetarian, pure and simple. And, as I mentioned, delicious. Think Raspberry Cheese Crumb Cake, Spinach and Portobello Mushroom Calzone, Golden Potato Chowder, Spicy Sesame Noodles, Grilled Vegetable Kebabs with Pecan Wild Rice, Baked Eggrolls with Sweet-Sour Sauce, and Double Chocolate Choco-Chip Cookies.

You *can* eat meat on occasion and still cash in on the power-up benefits of clearer, quicker thinking, better memory and concentration, improved creativity, more stable moods, less anxiety, greater calm, better endurance and strength, faster reaction time, greater agility, stronger immunity, reduced risk of disease, and more. But power-eating at its best revels in vegetarian cuisine.

Years ago, vegetarian cuisine was defined by what didn't show up on the plate: meat. Today it's a high-flavor, low-fat style of cooking in its own right. The finest chefs have made it trendy. For them, vegetarian cuisine means great taste. For us, it's great taste *and* the doorway to high performance of mind, mood, and body.

To help you take up the promise, this book offers the Power-Up Food Plan in three transition versions, menus, a list of smart lifestyle choices, endorphin-releasing exercise plans, answers to your power-up questions, and, of course, one-hundred-plus recipes.

The why, how, what, and when are all here. So is the who. You.

▪ HOW TO USE THIS BOOK ▪

I have divided *Energy Eating* into three parts: Why Power Up, How to Power Up, and Food and Recipes. You can read the book straight through or start with the chapters of greatest interest to you. If you endure PMS or the blues, for instance, you might want to turn immediately to chapter 3 to learn mood-enhancing techniques, then read the other chapters.

In many of the chapters you'll find Customizers. The Customizers enhance the core diet of my Power-Up Food Plan by outlining which foods to eat in abundance, when, and in what combinations for your specific nutrition needs. You determine your needs by scoring questionnaires. I urge you to pay close attention to these questionnaires and Customizers; they're indispensable to power-eating.

In part 2, you learn the Power-Up Food Plan, which is at the heart of *Energy Eating*. Rounding out part 2 are chapters on smart exercise, which I call "power-cise," and healthy lifestyle choices, aptly named "power-living." Following the recommendations can help you power up better and faster. An example: Get goofy! We're loath to admit it, but we like to get silly. We need to play. That's because play taps into the wonder-filled part of us that never grew up—and shouldn't.

In Food and Recipes of part 3, out go the well-worn appetizer-salad-entree-accompaniment-dessert categories. Instead, you'll find brain boosters, energizers, stress busters, mood enhancers, PMS soothers, body builders, immunity boosters, and memory managers. Tested and retested, the recipes are low in fat and sugar but big on nutrition and, most important, flavor. Lots of flavor.

My favorite: the Miracle Chocolate Chip Cookie (of course!) with a secret fat-busting ingredient.

Finally, in an afterword, I share some thoughts on spirit power. I struggled over including it. But for me to write about brain power, mood power, and body power without addressing spirit power made no sense. So I had to write it.

Indulge.

I

Why Power Up

Think of yourself as a kneading bowl,
a sacred temple,
filled with the dough of your life:
your potential, your gifts, your hopes
and dreams, possibilities,
all that you are and can be.

—MACRINA WIEDERKEHR

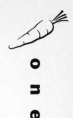

## one

How Food Powers Your Mind, Mood, and Body

You are what you eat. You eat what you are. These two simple sentences signal a profound truth, borne out by experience and backed by science: A new, healthier you—thanks to some amazing brain chemicals—is as close as your next meal.

Pioneering research into newly charted territories of the brain has discovered a treasure as valuable as all the gold in Fort Knox. It heralds the power-eating promise:

Eating the right foods at the right times in the right combinations can significantly boost your brain power, enhance your moods, and propel your physical performance to its peak.

In other words, a single meal can remake you, for better, for worse.

How so?

The latest research reveals that several crucial brain chemicals strongly influence your thinking abilities (including memory, concentration, and creativity), your moods, and your level of physical mastery. These brain chemicals are turned off and on by the foods you eat.

So when you take in brain-supporting foods, out comes mental clarity, better memory, contentment, energy, stronger immunity, and more. Much more.

You see, though the research already tells us a lot about how food turns on these amazing brain chemicals, in a few years researchers will share new discoveries. As we speak, hundreds of scientific studies on this very topic are under way. I have a hunch that the upcoming findings will taste as delicious as a ripe watermelon on a steamy July day, both figuratively and literally.

But there's no sense keeping secret the best research to date.

Energy Eating is the first book to pull together these latest research findings *and* disclose how to power-eat, power-cise, and power-live. You can't change your past, but you can choose your present. You can decide to think, feel, and perform at your highest God-given potential by making the most of what you've got.

The power-eating links to body and mind are becoming clearer, as you'll see as these chapters unfold. So, too, are the links to spirit. The medical community, which swallowed whole Rene Descartes's philosophy of the separateness of mind and body and soul (as did the rest of the Western world), is gradually recognizing the connectedness of the three.

While you boost brain power, enhance your mood, and achieve peak physical performance—and get in touch with God— you can power-eat to improve your looks too. Though this isn't a diet book, a welcome side effect of my Power-Up Food Plan (chapter 7) is bidding *adieu* to excess body fat.

Just the other day while rearranging my closet (I do crazy things like that before sitting down to write) I found my favorite jeans I wore in college nearly twenty years ago. I tried them on, curious if they still fit. They did indeed. In fact, my jeans fit better today than when I was nineteen. The difference: ten pounds of pudge from my abdomen, hips, and thighs.

Back in college, I lived for sausage pizza. Today I power-eat.

Simply put, power-eating is choosing foods to cause a desired effect. It pushes your biochemical hot buttons, rocketing your brain into a state of well-being where things click into place with ease. I call it the "Aha!" experience, when suddenly the light is turned on and you "see" as if for the first time and you go on an exhilarating mental-emotional-physical roll.

Food is more than nourishment. It's more than pleasure. It's your biochemical passport to the power-eating promise of tangible results *within minutes* of a meal. Yes, minutes. Not days, weeks, or months.

Consider this: Munching a high-protein snack like cheese on crackers raises the level of the amino acid tyrosine in your brain, boosting alertness.

Or this: When you eat a high-carbohydrate meal like spaghetti with marinara sauce, your body manufactures extra serotonin, a brain chemical, causing your stress level to drop.

Or this: Savoring a spinach soufflé, its main ingredients teeming with vitamin B_6 and choline, improves your ability to learn and remember.

And check out the long-term payoff of power-eating: reduced risk of

- many cancers
- arteriosclerosis
- stroke
- adult-onset diabetes
- osteoporosis
- obesity

Before we get to the "meat" of *Energy Eating,* a friendly word of advice: Please do consult your doctor or other health practitioner before following any recommendations on diet, dietary supplements, exercise, or stress reduction, especially if you are physically or mentally ill.

Though the recommendations in *Energy Eating* are backed by reams of the best science and can power up the lives of most of us, they won't cure depression or fatigue, leukemia, or other serious illnesses or conditions requiring medical care.

That said, let's recap a main point:

If you want to think your best . . .
If you want to feel your best . . .   *. . . Eat Your Best!*
If you want to perform your best . . .

For you to achieve the power-eating promise, you may think I'll recommend a bizarre eating regimen or a destined-to-fail fad diet. Not a chance. Power-eating is satisfying, for your mind, mood, and body—and your taste buds. It's as delicious as a watermelon on a hot summer day. You'll find a hundred-plus flavorful recipes in part 3, beginning on page 225.

But something is missing from these recipes, I confess: meat, with all of its saturated fat, cholesterol, and toxins, as well as one of the latest identified negatives—homocysteine, an amino acid that appears to be more dangerous to your health than cigarette smoking. The upshot: Regular meat-eating and power-eating are like oil and water. They don't mix.

Period.

▪ THE ULTIMATE DIET ▪

Step into a traditional kitchen on the picture-postcard island of Crete for an insider's view of the ingredients of power-eating. Piled on the tiled counters are the vibrant greens, purples, and reds of just-picked artichokes, fennel, peppers, spinach, eggplant, tomatoes, and beets and the yellows and oranges of citrus. Add in the rich browns of grains and legumes, from the palest beige to rusty brown-red to earthy black.

Now breathe in the fruity aroma of olive oil, used with a heavy hand, to America's fat-phobic mind-set. Smell the sweetness of roasted onions and garlic and fresh chives, mint, and cilantro. Taste the warmth of just-baked whole-grain bread.

Then listen to the music of a satisfied soul.

But where are the gyros? the moussaka? and all the other heavy foods I find in the restaurants of Greektown, one of my hometown Chicago's celebrated neighborhoods? You won't find them in a traditional kitchen of Crete, where simple is considered the best.

Oh, there may be some chicken in the icebox for a special occasion. But meat is only a small part of the flavorful Mediterranean diet. Eggs and milk? Not in this traditional kitchen. Cheese? Usually. Not cheddar or Monterey Jack, but hunks of goat cheese, a wonderfully mild and naturally lower-fat mainstay. In fact, foods of animal origin (meat, fish, eggs, and dairy products) account for a mere 7 percent of the traditional diet of Crete, where people live long and well.

The Cretans boast a health statistic that shames America and much of the Western world. Their rate of heart disease is about a tenth of that in the United States and other industrialized nations, and cancer is rare. This finding, which holds true to this day, was made in the sixties by the legendary epidemiologist Ancel Keys, who compared the longevity and the incidences of illness of different populations. His work helped indict dietary cholesterol and saturated fat, which, as you probably know, come to us primarily from meat.

■ ALL-TIME HIGH ■

Interest in vegetarian cuisine in America is at an all-time high as we enter the twenty-first century, despite the efforts of fad-diet peddlers who hawk high-protein, meat-centered diets. The best surveys to date indicate that twenty thousand adult Americans become vegetarian *each week*. If this pace keeps up, American vegetarians will number thirty million by the year 2010.

Many of these "new" vegetarians do not fit Webster's definition: a person who eats "wholly of vegetables [including grains, legumes, nuts, and seeds], fruits, and sometimes eggs or dairy products." I call them "almost vegetarians" or "alternavores." They recognize that the vegetarian diet is ideal, yet they want to have their occasional crab cake and eat it too. Their number-one reason to eat more like a vegetarian is health.

Though almost vegetarians can get results from my Power-Up Food Plan, which I'll describe in a moment and detail extensively in chapter 7, the ideal diet eliminates the meat, has a healthy amount of eggs and dairy products (though you can do well with none), and revels in every imaginable vegetable, fruit, grain, and legume.

It powers up your mind, mood, and body *effectively and deliciously.* Really, if it ain't delicious, why eat it?

Says top nutritionist Marion Nestle: "There's no question that largely vegetarian diets are as healthy as you can get. The evidence is so strong and overwhelming and produced over such a long period of time that it's no longer debatable."

For a picture of a power-eater, imagine Martina Navratilova charging the net, her muscles taut, poised to smash the ball, while her opponent shrinks in imminent defeat. Navratilova is undoubtedly the strongest female tennis player, physically and mentally, in the history of her sport.

Quite some time ago, she cut red meat out of her diet, hoping to improve her game, and she did. Then in the early nineties, Navratilova ended her love affair with chicken and other animal foods. She played and felt even better.

"I've noticed that I have an easier time getting going in the morning and a faster recovery after a tough workout," she told *Vegetarian Times,* where I was the executive editor and rubbed shoulders with vegetarian chefs and celebrities. When she retired from singles play in her late thirties, Navratilova was still racking up championships.

You, too, can quickly and effectively eat your way out of many food-related problems, whether your complaint is poor energy, the blues, poor concentration, anxiety, foggy memory, or less-than-best physical performance.

You just need a plan—the Power-Up Food Plan.

▪ WHAT'S THE POWER-UP FOOD PLAN? ▪

Before I describe what it is, let me tell you what it isn't. My Power-Up Food Plan is not a weight-loss diet, though you'll probably shed excess pounds almost effortlessly. It's not the secret to staying young forever, but it will rev up your immune system. It's not some funky New Age solution to finding your "power" within; the food itself is the God-given fuel for your mind, body, and spirit.

My Power-Up Food Plan is your ticket to thinking, feeling, and performing your very best. It has an icing-on-the-cake feature: a core diet (the "cake") with mini-plans called Customizers (the "icing"). Among them are the Blues-Buster Customizer, Anti-PMS Customizer, Super-Fit Customizer, and Live-Long Customizer.

For many people, the core satisfies. It has a scientifically sound profile of 10 to 15 percent of calories from protein, 60 to 70 percent from carbohydrates, and 20 to 25 percent from fat. It teems with antioxidants, B vitamins, calcium, iron, zinc, and other important nutrients. It specifies in detail which foods to eat in abundance and when.

Timing is crucial. For example, lunching on angel hair pasta topped with vegetables and a splash of olive oil, and a monster-size dish of frozen yogurt can be bad for your brain. This high-carbohydrate, low-protein meal might make you mentally sluggish. But this same meal at dinnertime can help you relax and let go of the cares of the day.

Energy Eating also has essential components on exercise and healthy lifestyle choices, dubbed power-cising and power-living, in chapters 8 and 9, respectively. This dynamic duo works in tandem with power-eating to elicit the coveted "Aha!" experience.

■ SCIENCE BACKS IT ■

For years, researchers have known that vegetarians succumb to fewer illnesses and live longer than people choosing meals weighed down by meat and its saturated fat, cholesterol, and toxins. That's reason enough to go green.

But then a most provocative scientific finding was unveiled

nearly thirty years ago: Eating certain foods affects brain chemistry and, in turn, your moods. What does this have to do with my Power-Up Food Plan?

Everything.

When you combine the latest discoveries in brain chemistry with the proven healthfulness of vegetarian cuisine, you reach the very heart of the power-eating promise.

Richard Wurtman, a neuroscientist at the Massachusetts Institute of Technology in Cambridge, made the initial discovery of how food affects brain chemistry. His research team fed rats mostly starch and sugar and found elevated serotonin levels in their brains. Serotonin is the "comforting" neurotransmitter, a brain chemical you'll be hearing a lot about in the pages to come.

Joining her husband in the research, Judith Wurtman, also an MIT scientist,

---

THE TRUTH ABOUT PROTEIN

The too-little-protein myth has dogged vegetarians for decades. Even today, one of the first questions I'm asked is, So where do you get your protein?

Let's settle this question once and for all: Getting enough protein is not a problem for vegetarians or almost vegetarians. So say dozens of research studies. Adding in its two cents, the conservative American Dietetic Association stated in its 1988, 1993, and 1997 position papers on vegetarian diets that vegetarians get *more* protein than they need.

The protein brouhaha flared up nearly thirty years ago when sociologist Frances Moore Lappé proposed the theory of protein complementarity, which urged vegetarians to mix and match foods that have different amino acid profiles to attain a "complete" protein.

While this theory sounds good on paper, the truth is you don't have to be so terribly careful. Even if you eat nothing but legumes, which are low in the amino acid methionine, for instance, you would not court a protein deficiency because the level of methionine is high enough to meet your protein needs.

Of course, no one ought to subsist on a single food. You need to eat sufficient calories from a variety of foods for overall health. Only people facing starvation or who have a rare metabolic disorder are at risk for protein deficiency.

Let's bury the too-little-protein myth once and for all.

---

soon became the undisputed leader of the mood-food movement. She has penned several books on the topic and developed a prepackaged, pure-carbohydrate drink mix for women with premenstrual syndrome. In the late 1990s, she told a standing-room only audience in Boston: "If a woman really has emotional pain, this drink will help her decrease her pain in fifteen to twenty minutes."

Such a claim from a highly respected scientist deserves a hearing, for it strongly suggests you are what you eat. And vice versa. What you savor at one meal or snack helps determine your food choices at the next meal.

Let's say you lunched on batter-dipped fried mushrooms, angel hair pasta tossed in olive oil and adorned with grilled vegetables, a dressed green salad, and a goblet of chocolate mousse. Within an hour or so, you will probably feel sluggish from your fat-heavy and low-protein lunch and will be tempted to plunk change into the vending machine for a candy bar. The sugar rush will boost your alertness for a short time, then your mood will spiral south, causing you to sneak some M&Ms from a candy dish or to find the nearest coffeepot for a caffeine quickie. You'll feel better again for a while, then crash again, prompting another round of bad food choices.

The Power-Up Plan shows you how to choose your meals wisely so you make it easy for yourself to eat right. A good meal "talks" to your brain cells, urging more good food. They willingly agree. It's power-eating at its best.

To feel, think, and perform your finest, you must provide the right fuel to an often overlooked part of your body: your nervous system.

■ YOU'VE GOT THE NERVE ■

You were born with 100 billion neurons, or brain cells, and you've lost about 100,000 neurons a day since then. You will continue to lose 100,000 neurons each day, leaving you with a little over 96 billion neurons at age one hundred, somewhat fewer if you abuse alcohol or drugs or endure chronic stress or illness.

Well-connected, each neuron is able to communicate with 1,000 to 6,000 other neurons, making about 100 trillion connections at any given moment. Chemical couriers known as neurotransmitters carry the messages from one neuron's transmitting axon to another neuron's receiving dendrite at a synapse.

A synapse is the tiny space between an axon and a dendrite where neurotransmitters are secreted. Each neuron has 1,000 to 500,000 synapses. The more synapses you have, the smarter you probably are. In fact, one definition of learning is the establishment of new synapses.

Every thought you have, every emotion you feel, and every move you make derives from the connections between neurons made by the all-important neurotransmitters. Neurotransmitters have been compared to letters of the alphabet, with their "words" corresponding to thoughts, feelings, and behaviors—everything from blinking an eye to crying to adding together numbers to making a birthday wish. Without neurotransmitters, neurons would have no way to talk to each other and brain function would cease.

IF YOU EAT MEAT . . .

You might wonder whether *Energy Eating* can boost your brain power, enhance your moods, and help you achieve peak physical performance.

The unequivocal answer: yes.

Now don't read me wrong. Savoring delicious and healthy vegetarian foods is the ideal because they're stuffed with vitamins, minerals, and phytochemicals and, even more important, they have a coveted mix of carbohydrates, protein, and fat. The meat-heavy fare typical of most Americans' plates has too much fat and protein and too little carbo-rich foods.

But eating an occasional chicken breast or grilled salmon steak won't kill you. In fact, the celebrated Mediterranean diet known for its healthfulness and good flavor includes animal food, but in small portions. Meat isn't at the center of the plate, but on the side; a complement to the meal, not its raison d'être.

So what's the best way to power-eat while enjoying a favorite meat dish now and then?

First, make peace with the fact that power-eating means cutting back on meat (beef, pork, poultry, fish, and seafood).

Second, learn some simple techniques of replacing meat with flavorful vegetarian cuisine:

- If you eat several meat-centered meals weekly, start by replacing a third to a half of them with vegetarian dishes. The recipes in part 3, beginning on page 225, are an excellent start.
- Reduce the amount of meat in some meals you still eat. For instance, if you usually make your favorite sauté with chicken, use only half the usual amount and add extra vegetables.
- When shopping for meat, choose lean, preferably organic cuts. Look in

natural food stores to find such meat, which comes from animals that have not been fed hormones, pesticide-laced feed, or antibiotics. Along the same lines, avoid fish and seafood from polluted waters.

- Eat meat wisely. Since it's fat-heavy, save it until later in the day (or have just a few tidbits at lunch) when you don't need all of the benefits of power-eating. Fat slows digestion and, thus, interferes with thinking, feeling, and performing at your highest potential. Avoid meat altogether when your mood needs the lift that carbos can give it.

Third, keep an open mind. As you notice the power-eating benefits of vegetarian cuisine, take the smart step of trying a week or two of vegetarian-only power meals. Don't be surprised if you feel so good that you eagerly join the ranks of the twenty thousand Americans who become vegetarians each week.

There are two broad categories of neurotransmitters: the excitatory, which cause a neuron to fire, and the inhibitory, which prevent firing. Whether to fire depends on a "vote" within a single neuron. When a neuron fires, the neurotransmitters pass a message to other neurons. In addition, the communications vary in strength, the same way you can alter the loudness of your voice. Taking into account all the possible strengths, the number of communications among neurons is beyond human comprehension. One scientist estimated it at roughly ten raised to the trillionth power.

Although much of the brain remains a mystery to scientists, so far they have discovered more than fifty neurotransmitters. The most common type are simple amino acids, the building blocks of protein molecules. But the ones we're most interested in are the catecholamines, which include norepinephrine and dopamine; the indoleamines, which include serotonin; acetylcholine; and the neuropeptides, which include endorphins, galanin, and neuropeptide Y.

For an idea of how a meal figures in, let's look at serotonin, dopamine, and norepinephrine.

Say that you're jittery and want to calm down. Serotonin, often called the "comforting" neurotransmitter, is manufactured from the amino acid tryptophan found in protein foods. Ironically, eating protein does not increase tryptophan levels. The trick is to eat carbohydrates (or *carbos* for short) such as potatoes, bread, grains, soft drinks, and candy. In an indirect chain of events, when you choose a carbo, your brain level of tryptophan increases, triggering a rise in serotonin. Within thirty minutes your jitters will probably diminish.

low serotonin → bad mood (including the jitters) → desire for carbos → eat carbos → increase of brain tryptophan → increase of serotonin → improved mood

Now let's pretend you've got a test in a hour and you feel mentally sluggish. Hello, dopamine and norepinephrine, the "alertness" neurotransmitters, which are synthesized from tyrosine, an amino acid supplied best by foods of animal origin (dairy products and eggs as well as meat), legumes, nuts, and seeds. Nibble on a wedge of low-fat cheese and your brain level of tyrosine goes up, as do your dopamine and norepinephrine if they were low. Very soon you may feel mentally agile and are better able to handle a stress.

mental sluggishness → desire for protein → eat protein food → increase of brain tyrosine → increase of dopamine and norepinephrine → brain power boost

Here's a curious twist: Whenever you eat protein (the type doesn't matter) tyrosine will reach your brain even if you also eat a high-carbo food. But for comforting tryptophan to get to your brain, you must eat carbos alone.

How come? Tyrosine, tryptophan, and four other amino acids all enter the brain on a common highway, so to speak. Because space is limited, all of these neurotransmitters cannot speed into the brain at once.

Think of it this way: The competing amino acids are cars circulating in your blood vessels. The "tryptophan" model is the least common, allowing greater numbers of the other cars onto the ramps leading to the highway to the brain. The only way for tryptophan cars to enter the highway is for the other cars to stay off. For this to happen, you must eat carbos alone.

Carbohydrates trigger the release of the hormone insulin from the pancreas. Insulin behaves like a police vehicle, causing amino acids other than tryptophan to pull over into various body cells. With tyrosine and the other amino acids out of the way, the tryptophan cars can flood the ramps leading to the highway to the brain.

▪ THE POWER-UP NEUROTRANSMITTERS ▪

Via the neurotransmitters, your brain can effectively communicate what it needs for optimal functioning. Here's a look at ones that figure in to power-eating.

Serotonin: This "comforting" neurotransmitter is released after eating carbos alone. When your serotonin brain levels are low, you feel blue, irritable, anxious, moody, or a similar negative emotion. At a biochemical level, your body deeply desires starch (bread, pasta, potatoes) or sugar (fruit, sweet baked goods, desserts) to balance your bad mood.

Norepinephrine: Manufactured from protein foods, this neurotransmitter, which is also called noradrenaline, regulates mental functioning such as alertness and your ability to think quickly and accurately and to cope with stress. A low level of noradrenaline is also associated with depression. So when you need energy and a mental tune-up, eat protein with or without carbos but never eat carbos alone.

Dopamine: This neurotransmitter goes hand in hand with norephinephrine, behaving much the same way.

Acetylcholine: This neurotransmitter is synthesized from choline, a fatlike substance abundant in eggs and wheat germ. It's your body's memory manager. When acetylcholine levels dwindle, which is common during chronic stress and in aging, your ability to remember wanes, as does your overall cognitive functioning. Alzheimer's disease includes a loss of acetylcholine receptors, by the way.

Endorphins: These morphinelike chemicals send pleasure signals throughout the body. They boost your tolerance to pain, calm you when you're stressed, and produce feelings of satisfaction. Some research suggests eating fat and sugar may produce endorphins. Your best bet for an endorphin rush is chocolate. But don't overdo it: Chocolate contains anandamide, the body's own version of the active ingredient in marijuana, thus multiplying the pleasurable effects of this food; eating too much may actually create a physiological addiction.

Neuropeptide Y: Called NPY for short, this neurotransmitter turns on your appetite for carbos. It's jump-started by waning blood-sugar levels brought on by low glycogen stores in the liver and muscles. Your stores drop during the night while you're sleeping, so in the morning, NPY sends the message: Pig out on carbos. No wonder we often choose cereal, bagels, pancakes, waffles, and oatmeal for breakfast. Stress and strict dieting also trigger NPY production.

Galanin: This neuropeptide is the other major appetite-stimulating neurotransmitter. Higher levels of galanin increase your desire for fat. Galanin increases in the body when several hours have passed between meals. It's a survival chemical, safeguarding your body's fat.

NPY and galanin play a role in determining what you eat and thus your mood. They teeter-totter throughout the day.

■ THE POWER-UP NUTRIENTS ■

Your neurotransmitters cannot work alone to power your mind, mood, and body. They require helpers in their manufacture. The most important helpers are vitamins and minerals. For instance, without ample B vitamins, folic acid, vitamin C, and magnesium, your body won't make sufficient amounts of neurotransmitters. What's more, studies are showing that subtle deficiencies of various nutrients may further impair brain functioning.

A yardstick for measuring your needs is the Recommended Dietary Allowances (RDAs), which are the levels of intake of essential nutrients considered to be adequate to meet the known nutritional needs of practically all persons, according to the Food and Nutrition Board of the National Academy of Sciences, which formulated the RDAs.

A snafu: The RDAs are meant to help healthy people avoid severe deficiency diseases, like beriberi, which are rare in Western nations. They aren't designed for people desiring optimal functioning. Not only that, common daily stresses (like driving at rush hour or keeping up with your toddler) can increase nutritional needs, as do poor eating and lifestyle habits, such as a sugar-laden diet and smoking.

This is why many people need supplements, particularly antioxidants like beta-carotene and vitamins C and E. Experts say safe and effective daily amounts of these antioxidants are 10 to 20 milligrams for beta-carotene, 250 to 1,000 milligrams for vitamin C, and 100 to 400 International Units (IU) for vitamin E.

With the exceptions of vitamins A and D (which are toxic in large doses), you can safely take up to double the RDAs of the other vitamins and minerals, and even 1 to 2 grams of vitamin C daily and 800 IU of vitamin E daily. (See "Do You Need a Supplement?" page 132.)

Even power-eaters may need supplements, especially when calorie intake dips below 2,000 calories a day, with chronic stress or the use of tobacco or other drugs (including coffee).

Here's a rundown of the helpers by category. If you are pregnant or lactating, your needs increase; consult your doctor or other health practitioner.

■ THE PERKY B VITAMINS ■

You want B's on your nutrition report card. They are critical to the manufacturing of neurotransmitters. In addition, depression, poor energy, and reduced mental functioning have been linked to inadequate levels.

	WHAT IT DOES	RDA	SOURCES
Vitamins B_1 (thiamin) and B_2 (riboflavin)	Critical to synthesis of acetylcholine.	B_1: 1.1mg for females 11+ yrs.; 1.3 to 1.5mg for males 11+ yrs. B_2: 1.3mg for females 11+ yrs.; 1.5 to 1.8mg for males 11+ yrs.	B_1: rice bran, wheat germ, legumes, Brazil nuts, soy foods, pine nuts, green peas, whole-grain flour, tahini. B_2: yogurt, cottage cheese, almonds, milk, ricotta cheese, wheat germ, cheese.
Vitamin B_3 (niacin)	Works with B_1 and B_2 in facilitating energy production in cells. A deficiency leads to a condition known as pellagra, marked by the malfunctioning of the nervous system. The body can convert the amino acid tryptophan into niacin.	15mg for females 11+ yrs.; 17 to 20mg for males 11+ yrs.	Eggs, whole grains, nuts, legumes.
Vitamin B_5	Known as pantothenic acid. Is converted to co-enzyme A, important in the synthesis of the neurotransmitter acetylcholine.	No RDA. Suggested: 4 to 7mg for individuals 11+ yrs.	Eggs, broccoli, milk, sweet potato, molasses, corn, lentils, peanuts, pecans, soy foods, sunflower seeds, wheat germ, whole-grain flour, blue cheese.

	WHAT IT DOES	RDA	SOURCES
Vitamin B_6	Necessary for serotonin production and for the metabolism of the amino acids used by the brain to manufacture neurotransmitters involved in mental energy and memory.	1.4 to 1.6mg for females 11+ yrs.; 1.7 to 2mg for males 11+ yrs.	Avocados, bananas, wheat and rice bran, carrots, filberts, lentils, rice, soy, wheat germ, leafy greens, whole-grain flour.
Folate (folic acid)	Helps manufacture serotonin, dopamine, and norepinephrine. A deficiency may lower serotonin levels and cause mood disorders.	80mcg for women 15+ yrs.; 200mcg for men 15+ yrs.	Barley, legumes, endive, fruits, leafy greens, rice, soy foods, sprouts, wheat germ.
Vitamin B_{12}	A general nervous system booster. Helps synthesize dopamine and norepinephrine from the amino acid tyrosine and serotonin from the amino acid tryptophan. A deficiency may lead to depression and memory problems.	2mcg for individuals 11+ yrs.	Eggs, dairy products, fortified cereal, fortified soymilk.

■ THE SUPER ANTIOXIDANTS ■

Antioxidants disarm free radicals, highly reactive molecules with unpaired electrons, which can damage your body's cells. Free radicals have been implicated in cancer, heart disease, and a host of other illnesses.

	WHAT IT DOES	RDA	SOURCES
Beta-carotene	The precursor to vitamin A, beta-carotene protects the nervous system.	For vitamin A, 800mcgRE for females 11+ yrs.; 1,000mcgRE for males 11+ yrs.	Pumpkin, sweet potato, carrot, mango, spinach, papaya, cantaloupe, kale, apricots, collards, tomato, asparagus.
Vitamin C	Protects nerve cells from damage by free radicals and helps in the manufacturing of acetylcholine and norepinephrine.	60mg for individuals 15+ yrs.	Papaya, guava, strawberries, kiwifruit, cantaloupe, broccoli, Brussels sprouts, grapefruit, cauliflower, potato, pineapple, cabbage, tomato, blueberries, sweet peppers, leafy greens.
Vitamin E	The most powerful antioxidant nutrient. Also protects beta-carotene from being destroyed in the body.	8mg for females 11+ yrs.; 10mg for males 15+ yrs.	Vegetable oils, almonds, filberts, walnuts, wheat germ, whole grains.
Selenium	Protects neurotransmitters from damage by free radicals. A low intake may bring on depression.	No RDA. Suggested: 0.05 to 0.2mg for individuals 7+ yrs.	Wheat and rice bran, broccoli, cabbage, celery, cucumbers, eggs, fresh garlic, milk, cheese, yogurt, mushrooms, onion, wheat germ, whole grains.

■ Feel-Good Minerals ■

Eating too few mineral-rich foods can cause depression, anxiety, irritability, and low energy, studies are showing. I've listed the ones you ought not to miss. If you're already taking in optimal amounts, getting more won't give you an extra boost.

	WHAT IT DOES	RDA	SOURCES
Magnesium	Necessary for the manufacture of dopamine and norepinephrine. A marginal intake is associated with depression.	280mg for females 19+ yrs.; 350mg for males 19+ yrs.;	Leafy greens, almonds, cashews, soy foods, seeds, dairy products, avocados, apples, apricots, figs, peaches, beets, whole grains.
Calcium	Eases PMS. Low intakes may cause poor mood, including depression.	800mg for individuals 25+ yrs.	Milk, yogurt, cheese, fortified orange juice, collards, figs, tofu made with calcium salts, spinach, broccoli, okra, amaranth, blackstrap molasses.
Iron	Too little iron can cause fatigue and depression.	15mg for females 11 to 50 yrs.; 10mg for older females and males 19+ yrs.	Legumes, sea vegetables, quinoa, spinach, bran cereal, figs, pumpkin seeds, sesame seeds, Swiss chard, lima beans, molasses, prunes, raisins, bulgur, apricots, wholewheat bread.

	WHAT IT DOES	RDA	SOURCES
Potassium	Helps maintain water balance. Also highly important in nerve transmission.	No RDA. Suggested: 2,000mg for adults.	Orange juice, bananas, dried fruits, bran, peanut butter, legumes, potatoes.
Zinc	Critical for some enzymatic reactions. Also important for insulin activity, protein synthesis, and immune function.	12mg for females 11+ yrs.; 15mg for males 11+ yrs.	Bran, egg yolks, blackstrap molasses, soy foods, sunflower seeds, wheat germ, whole grains.
Boron	Important in calcium and bone metabolism, possibly preventing bone loss associated with osteoporosis. May aid muscle-building by raising testosterone levels in men and women.	No RDA.	Soy foods, prunes, raisins, peanuts, hazelnuts.

■ Is Fat That Bad? ■

Yes and no.

Yes, hundreds of studies have implicated dietary fat in horrible illnesses like heart disease and some cancers. The fat you eat also affects your blood cholesterol levels and triglyceride levels. And, studies show, too much fat interferes with how well you think, feel, and perform. It can even cause impotence.

But, no, fat isn't the demon the media has portrayed it as.

Nearly fifteen years ago, says the Food Marketing Institute, only 16 percent of American consumers worried about the amount of fat in their diets. By 1995, 65 percent had the fat jitters. Consequently, the average American started eating less fat. Her fat intake dropped to 34 percent in the late nineties, down from 40 percent in 1977.

Yet the average American is plumper. You see, while fat intake dropped, the number of total calories in the diet zoomed higher. The fat-phobes jammed their shopping carts with low-fat and fat-free items, which are usually loaded with sugar to improve flavor and are hefty in calories. They shoveled in the sugar and gained weight.

All of this might seem an interesting twist of fate if it weren't for a serious flaw: Not all types of fat are harmful to you. Despite the official advice to cut back on all fats, the real devils are saturated fat and trans fatty acids.

As you probably know, saturated fat weighs down red meat, chicken, butter, whole milk, whole yogurt, full-fat cheeses, coconut oil, and palm kernel oil. A rule of thumb: If the fat is solid at room temperature, it's saturated.

Trans fatty acids are the new dangerous fats that mess up your body and mind. This type is at least as harmful to you as saturated fat, and maybe more so. Scientists continue to measure up its nasty nature.

At the risk of oversimplification, I'll describe trans fatty acids as twisted molecules made during food processing. They do not appear in nature. Considering how dangerous they are, you'd think that food labels would disclose their presence. Not so.

The new and improved food labels lump trans fatty acids with the polyunsaturated fats. That's because trans fatty acids are made from polyunsaturates. A polyunsaturated fat like soybean oil can be hydrogenated to make it a solid or semisolid fat. During the hydrogenation process, trans fatty acids are formed.

The best way to determine if a food product has trans fatty acids is by looking at the ingredient list. The tip-off: The words "hydrogenated" or "partially hydrogenated" mean trans fatty acids are probably lurking inside.

While it's smart to eat fewer saturated fats and trans fatty acids, researchers have not yet found much evidence that the other two types of fats—polyunsaturated and mono-unsaturated—are bad for you. In fact, they might have health benefits.

Remember the traditional kitchen we visited on the island of Crete? Not only do the people of Crete feast on delicious, heart-healthy, and brain-boosting food, they do so using lots of olive oil. The fat content of their diet ranges from 25 to 40 percent of calories.

The epidemiologist Ancel Keys found that the fat in olive oil, which is mostly monounsaturated, did not raise their overall blood cholesterol levels or jeopardize their health. Recent evidence suggests that polyunsaturates and monounsaturates may "dissolve" some of the saturates in your body and increase high-density lipoproteins (the "good" cholesterol).

Why am I giving you these fat facts?

Because in the confusion created by some diet docs pushing a cuisine of deprivation (with only 10 percent of calories from fat) while

---

A TOO SWEET PROBLEM

Ever hear of insulin resistance?

A best-seller of the midnineties made some wild claims about its prevalence, striking fear in the hearts of many a reader of the book and providing the media with a juicy story. While insulin resistance exists, the best research indicates it's a problem for about 25 percent of the American population.

Even one in four is a big number. However, if you're at a healthy weight, or maybe just five or ten pounds over, it's highly unlikely you have insulin resistance, because it targets the obese almost exclusively.

So what is it?

Insulin resistance is a condition that causes the hormone insulin to behave poorly. When an insulin-resistant person eats a meal, her pancreas overreacts to compensate for the insulin's inefficiency. Instead of increasing its secretion of insulin gradually and leveling off, the pancreas pumps out a ton of insulin, causing the levels to skyrocket and stay elevated for longer than normal.

The more often this happens, and the longer your insulin level remains high, the more likely you will overeat, because elevated insulin levels arouse the appetite. In addition, a high insulin level increases fat storage and inhibits the release of fat from your body's adipose tissues, or fat stores. So you store more fat and burn less stored fat.

The propensity toward insulin resistance may be partially genetic. But many insulin-resistant people can fight back.

The best method may be increasing fiber intake. Research indicates that eating fiber-rich foods improves the sensitivity and efficiency of insulin, so less insulin is needed to bring blood sugar to your body cells. Higher fiber means more fruits, vegetables, grains, and legumes and less dairy products and meat.

In a word, power-eat.

other self-proclaimed "experts" are saying steak every day is okay, you need the proof that the middle ground is the place to be. Especially when you want to maximize the way you think, feel, and perform.

My Power-Up Food Plan has 20 to 25 percent of calories from fat. That's more than enough for great taste at every meal and snack but not enough to interfere with optimal brain functioning.

As you'll hear in more detail in the next chapter, power-eating goes easy on fat for this important reason: Fat slows down and blunts the feel-good effects of neurotransmitters.

■ LIVING BETTER FOREVER ■

Before we go further, I must make a confession: I love chocolate. Chocolate chip cookies, chocolate chip ice cream, chocolate-covered cherries, and, most especially, foil-wrapped chocolate kisses. I keep a stash of kisses in a crystal jar on top of a cabinet far from the reach of my children.

Each day I unwrap a few of the kisses like presents, pop them in my mouth one at a time, and let them melt. Inside I glow. My neurons dance. Ah, heaven, pure heaven.

And no guilt. Not even a twinge.

You see, my research uncovered a delicious surprise: Chocolate is good for you. In moderation, that is. Scientists have found that chocolate contains phenolics, potent antioxidants that protect against heart disease, and other chemicals, like anandamide, that lift spirits. Its fat isn't the dangerous type, either. Three separate studies published in 1994 came to that conclusion.

So I indulge, but I don't go overboard. Too much of anything can be unhealthy. And so it is with eating chocolate. Or dieting. Or exercise.

This brings me to the absolute advantage of power-eating. It need not, and ought not, consume you. If you make poor food choices at one meal, you can do better at the next. Your reward for eating the right foods at the right times in the right combinations is almost immediate: the "Aha!" experience.

Thank your neurotransmitters. And thank heavens for *Theobroma cacao.*

Theo-what? *Theobroma cacao,* the scientific name of chocolate, means "the food of the gods."

Sounds heavenly to my endorphins.

POWER QUIZ

How Well Do You Eat Now?

You can't see the forest for the trees unless you back up and get a panoramic view. So it goes with your current eating style. This self-assessment surveys your strengths and your weaknesses, so you know which changes are best for you.

Circle the letter that most approximates the way you eat now.

1. How often do you eat vegetarian meals and snacks (which, by definition, contain no red meat, poultry, or fish)?

   a) at all meals and snacks   b) at 4 out of 5
   c) at 3 out of 5   d) at fewer than 3 out of 5

2. How often do you eat beef, veal, and pork?

   a) never   b) a few times a month
   c) several times a week   d) daily or almost daily

3. How often do you eat poultry and/or fish?

   a) never or infrequently   b) about once a week
   c) several times a week   d) daily or almost daily

4. How many meals and snacks do you eat daily?

   a) 5 or 6   b) 4   c) 3   d) less than 3

5. How many glasses of water do you drink daily?

   a) at least 7   b) 5 or 6   c) 3 or 4   d) less than 3

6. About how many calories do you eat daily?

   a) at least 2,500 (for men and active women) or 2,200 (for other women)
   b) 2,100 to 2,400 (for men and active women) or 1,800 (for other women)
   c) 1,800 to 2,000 (for men and active women) or 1,500 (for other women)
   d) less than 1,700 (for men and active women) or less than 1,200 (for other women)

7. How close is your weight to what's ideal for you?

   a) close to ideal
   b) about 10 pounds over-weight
   c) more than 15 pounds underweight
   d) at least 20 percent over ideal

8. How many servings of grains do you eat daily?

   a) at least 8
   b) 6 or 7
   c) 4 or 5
   d) fewer than 4

9. How many of your grain servings come from whole sources, such as whole-wheat bread or brown rice?

   a) all or almost all
   b) half
   c) a third
   d) fewer than a third

10. How many vegetable servings do you eat daily?

    a) at least 4
    b) 3
    c) 2
    d) 1 or 0

11. How often do you have a serving of dark leafy greens, such as spinach, chard, or kale?

    a) every day
    b) several times a week
    c) occasionally
    d) almost never

12. How many fruit servings do you eat daily?

    a) at least 3
    b) 2
    c) 1
    d) less than 1

13. How often do you have a serving of a vitamin C–rich vegetable or fruit?

    a) at least twice a day   b) once a day
    c) several times a week   d) occasionally

14. How often do you have a serving of a beta-carotene–rich vegetable or fruit?

    a) at least twice a day   b) once a day
    c) several times a week   d) occasionally

15. How many legume servings do you eat weekly?

    a) at least 6   b) 4 or 5   c) 2 or 3   d) less than 2

16. How many servings of nuts and seeds do you eat weekly?

    a) 8 to 14   b) 5 to 7   c) 2 to 4   d) less than 2

17. How many servings of dairy foods or high-calcium plant foods do you eat?

    a) 2 a day   b) 1 a day
    c) several each week   d) very few a week

18. How often do you have a serving of eggs (including eggs in baked goods)?

    a) a few times each week   b) 1 or 2 times each week
    c) at least once a day   d) never

19. What is the fat percentage of your total daily caloric intake?

    a) 20 to 25 percent   b) 25 to 30 percent
    c) less than 20 percent   d) over 30 percent

20. How often do you eat refined sugar and/or products in which refined sugar is a primary ingredient?

    a) rarely
    b) occasionally
    c) at least once a day
    d) several times a day

21. How often do you eat a healthy breakfast, like oatmeal with raisins, high-fiber, low-sugar cold cereal with milk, or waffles or pancakes with fruit spread?

    a) every day
    b) almost every day
    c) a few times a week
    d) rarely

22. Which most closely decribes your typical snack?

    a) a couple of pieces of fruit
    b) a bagel
    c) fruited yogurt
    d) cookies or chips

23. How much caffeine do you take in daily?

    a) very little or none
    b) about 40 milligrams (the amount in a five-ounce cup of tea)
    c) about 100 milligrams (the amount in a five-ounce cup of coffee)
    d) more than 100 milligrams

24. How many servings of alcohol do you have? (A serving is equal to five ounces of wine, twelve ounces of beer, or one ounce of liquor.)

    a) 0 to 1 a day
    b) 0 to 1 a week, or fewer
    c) 1 to 2 a day
    d) more than 2 a day

25. How often do you limit your intake of salt and salty foods?

    a) almost always
    b) usually
    c) fairly often
    d) seldomly

26. How many weight-reducing diets have you tried in your life-
    time?

    a) no more than 2   b) 3 or 4
    c) about 5   d) too many to count

27. How often do you take a moderate-dose vitamin and mineral
    supplement?

    a) daily   b) several times a week
    c) several times a month   d) never

---

*For each "a" you circled give yourself one point; for each "b" two
points; for each "c" three points; and for each "d" four points.
Then tally your score. The lowest possible score is 27 while the
highest is 108.*

27 to 40 points: Excellent! You're well on the road to power-
eating. Look over your marks and decide to improve in areas
where you circled a *c* or *d*.

41 to 55: Pretty good, but you have room to improve. First work
on improving your *d* marks, then the *c*'s.

56 to 70: Average. While you may have a number of *d*'s and *c*'s,
be encouraged: This book will tell you how and why to choose a
healthier eating style.

71 and over: Yikes! Read this book tonight and start making the
very doable, painless changes tomorrow—or sooner.

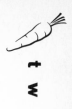

Boosting Your Brain Power

"At lunch, I almost always eat light," my attorney friend Carolyn confided. "When I eat a big lunch or a fatty lunch, I am mentally sluggish all afternoon. That's bad for business. When I eat a light lunch, I stay alert. I feel so much better. I think so much better."

Carolyn power-eats. She began power-eating three years ago, trading in red meat and other fatty foods for grains, vegetables, and fruits, with an occasional fish supper, and eating them at the right times in the right combinations. She lost weight but was more impressed with what she gained: mental agility, clearer and quicker thinking, improved concentration, and better memory. In two words, brain power.

To quickly gauge your brain power, answer these questions:

1. When writing reports for work or school, do the perfect words pop in your head faster than you can type them?

   _____ *Often* _____ *Sometimes* _____ *Rarely*

2. Do you design, organize, decorate, sculpt, or paint with a Picasso-like creativity?

   _____ *Often* _____ *Sometimes* _____ *Rarely*

3. Have you attended office picnics or neighborhood block parties and remembered everyone's name (even the spouses' and kids' names)?

_____ *Often*   _____ *Sometimes*   _____ *Rarely*

If you circled *often* or *sometimes,* you've experienced the wonder of brain power. Some people call it a mental roll; I call it the "Aha!" experience: those moments when things click into place, like a light switch being turned on, as neurons zoom messages to one another with speed and perfection, making you feel like the smartest person on Earth.

All in all, the research shows that power-eating is your meal ticket to charging up your brain. Exercise helps tremendously too. So do intelligent lifestyle choices. (See chapters 8 and 9.)

Eating the right foods at the right times in the right combinations won't make you smarter than you are. But you'll think your best because you'll make the most of what you've got.

Equally wonderful, brain power is within your grasp every day.

Waltz into your kitchen and you'll be surrounded by brain-power foods. And by brain-drain foods. You just need to know which are which—and why. In my wellness counseling, I've noticed that when people know why foods profoundly affect their minds, moods, and bodies, they're far more likely to make power-up choices.

Think tyrosine.

■ THE BRAINY PROTEIN ■

Tyrosine is your gateway to brain power. It's an amino acid that comes with lunch. Actually, *in* lunch. Although tyrosine, a building block of protein, fills many foods, it can be wiped out of your bloodstream by a heavy dose of carbohydrates.

First, let's look at the two ways tyrosine gets from your food to your brain, triggering the manufacture of the "alertness" neurotransmitters, namely, norepinephrine and dopamine.

As mentioned in the previous chapter, neurotransmitters are biochemical messengers that pass important chunks of information from one neuron (brain cell) to another. The neurotransmitters we're most interested in are serotonin, acetylcholine, the endorphins, and the catecholamines, which include norepinephrine and dopamine.

Tyrosine is the precursor to norepinephrine and dopamine, and its best suppliers are protein-rich foods like legumes, nuts, and seeds, and foods of animal origin (dairy products, eggs, and, yes, meat).

When you eat one of these foods with or without carbohydrates, your blood level of tyrosine rises. As tyrosine goes up, so do your levels of norepinephrine and dopamine *if* they were low to begin with. Some researchers say your levels of norepinephrine and dopamine drop to brain-impairing levels only in times of extreme stress, say, hand-to-hand combat during war or a ten-mile hike in the Antarctic. Other researchers contend that the stress of driving in rush-hour traffic is enough to fiddle with your levels of these neurotransmitters.

low stores of norepinephrine and dopamine → eat protein food → increase of tyrosine levels → increase of norepinephrine and dopamine → brain power boost

The second way to a mental roll: Never, ever overdose on carbos by eating them alone.

Eating platefuls of pasta for lunch can make you fuzzy-headed. That's because a high-carbo meal without any protein paves the way for the amino acid tryptophan to flood your brain. From tryptophan, your brain manufactures serotonin, the "comforting" neurotransmitter that can make you sleepy, slow, and mentally exhausted.

My friend Jennifer, a schoolteacher, experienced the tryptophan slowdown the day I counseled her. A vegetarian for nearly four years, Jennifer had savored whole-wheat bread, a baked potato with nonfat sour cream, and strawberries for lunch that day.

"I was calm going into lunch," Jennifer said. "But I left school feeling mentally drained."

To recap, if you eat carbos alone when you're calm, relaxed, content, or tired, you're setting up a brain drain.

calm or tired mood → eat carbos alone → increase of tryptophan levels → increase of serotonin → brain drain (i.e., fuzzy-headedness, dull thinking, poor concentration, mental lethargy)

The hormone insulin takes the credit (or blame, depending on how you see it) for allowing the manufacture of serotonin. When you eat carbos alone, your pancreas releases insulin into the bloodstream, causing tyrosine and four other amino acids to scoot from your blood into various body cells while tryptophan speeds into your brain.

Truly, insulin is one of the most interesting hormones in your body. In fact, the authors of several fad diet books of the mid-nineties pounced on insulin's role in achieving ideal weight, pushed a meat-heavy, low-carbohydrate diet, and sold millions of copies. As we revisit insulin and brain power throughout this chapter, you'll see the truth.

▪ A BRAIN DRAINER ▪

Eating too much fat, and especially saturated fat in meat, dulls your brain.

How so?

As we heard from Carolyn, who, you remember, stopped eating fatty lunches, a fat feast slows your digestion dramatically. Your body diverts blood away from your brain and to your digestive tract to handle the load.

As a glucose addict, your brain slurps up blood sugar. When well nourished, your brain is like a kid in a candy store, alert, eager, ready to act fast. But your brain takes a nap when your body busies itself with metabolizing fat globules. You can't think quickly or learn, remember, or concentrate well. And your creativity sinks into the pits.

Likewise, a high-calorie meal (more than 1,000 calories)—even if it's not loaded with fat—can make you mentally sluggish. A study from the University of Wales compared the thinking abilities of thirty-five women who ate one of three lunches: normal-sized, high-calorie (40 percent over their individual energy needs), and low-calorie (40 percent under their individual energy needs). The results: The women who ate the high-calorie lunch made the most errors on attention tests and search tasks.

Research indicates that the best eating schedule for most people is breakfast-snack-lunch-snack-dinner, with no single meal or snack exceeding 500 or so calories. To show the mental boost of snacking, scientists at Tufts University gave late-afternoon goodies (candy or yogurt) to college-aged men and measured their cognitive performance on a variety of tests. After the yogurt snack, the men solved significantly more arithmetic problems in less time than after eating the candy. But after either snack, the men recalled more digits and responded faster in an attention task than when they had a caffeine-free diet soda without a snack.

Dieting is another brain drainer. In one study, fifty-five dieters, aged eighteen to forty, scored poorly on a mental aptitude test compared to nondieters. Dieting also can induce sugar cravings, which interfere with thinking abilities.

The best way to lose weight and stay mentally sharp is to cut some fat out of your meals and lose pounds very gradually, about two pounds a month.

The bottom line: Eating too much fat can be downright dumb. And that's exactly why the Power-Up Food Plan contains a healthy amount of healthy fats.

■ HOW SWEET IT ISN'T ■

Your brain weighs only three pounds—about 2 percent of your body's total weight—but devours 20 percent of your total energy supply and close to 30 percent of the oxygen you breathe in. It depends on glucose to feed its millions of daily thought processes made possible by neurotransmitters.

Glucose is your body's favorite sugar. When you eat complex carbohydrates like bread, pasta, potatoes, and rice or simple carbohydrates like lactose in milk or sucrose in a sugar cube, your body turns them into mostly glucose molecules. (Fructose in fruit always enters your metabolism as fructose, however.) You'll see how in a moment.

If it exhausts its stores of glucose in the liver and muscles, your body is forced to run on fat and protein—a potentially dangerous situation.

Without the presence of carbohydrates, fats burn inefficiently and produce ketones (waste products). When your blood becomes polluted with ketones, your brain cannot function well. You may feel mentally and physically fatigued. Your kidneys, too, are overtaxed. They have the job of clearing ketones from your blood.

When your body must rely on protein for energy, this vital nutrient is less available for its essential functions of building and repairing tissues, which is more bad news for your brain. What's more, your immune system can't function as well, possibly making your brain prey to Alzheimer's disease and other age-related illnesses.

Clearly, carbos are key.

But which are best for powering up your brain? The starches (complex carbohydrates) or the sugars (simple carbohydrates)?

It's no contest: The starches win hands down.

To digest starches, a series of enzymes go to work. Over two hours, assuming you ate a low-fat meal, these enzymes break down the long, complex starch molecules into disaccharides. Then, in the walls of the small intestine, these are broken down into monosaccharides, including glucose. The single glucose molecules are readily absorbed into the body and first go to the liver, where some are stored and the rest are released into the bloodstream. (Glucose is sometimes called "blood sugar.")

A slow and steady fuel, starch is exactly what your brain

requires for optimal functioning. The glucose molecules enter your bloodstream gradually, prompting a healthy, moderate increase in your insulin level.

Sugar, in contrast, quickly boosts blood sugar and you feel a rush of energy. However, your insulin level is also boosted, and soon your blood sugar level plummets and your brain bonks.

Here's how it works: A simple carbohydrate like glucose has a short chain, with only two molecules per chain. Simple to digest and absorb, a simple carbohydrate needs only one of four enzymes to break the chain, a task completed in almost no time. Glucose molecules zip into your bloodstream via the liver.

That's bad news. You see, when you eat sugar, your pancreas dumps insulin

> **THE SUGAR BOOGIE BLUES**
>
> Eating sweets may invite the dance of sugar boogie, dampening brain power, mood power, and body power. Here's how the steps go.
>
> First, you eat a candy bar or drink a soda pop.
>
> Then your blood glucose level leaps and you feel energized.
>
> Next, the hormone insulin jumps in and bounces the glucose molecules into your body cells. But because insulin does such a good job, your blood glucose level dips, very fast and very far.
>
> Now your glucose-hungry brain chants, "More sugar, now." Your brain chemicals oblige. You get a sugar craving, and indulge once again.
>
> And so the boogie continues—until you stop it.
>
> The best way is to "just say no" to sugary foods in the first place. But if you have a biological craving for, say, chocolate, go ahead and have a little. It's fine to eat sweets now and then, but choose moderate amounts and eat them with complex carbohydrates, protein, and a little fat to blunt sugar's effect on your insulin level.
>
> For instance, precede your chocolate mousse with a power dinner of black bean burritos, a salad of kiwifruit, oranges, and jicama, and cinnamon tea.
>
> And do the sugar boogie no more.

into your bloodstream to regulate blood sugar. The insulin ushers glucose molecules into your body cells. And for a few glorious moments, your brain is on a sugar high.

Then comes the crash, as detrimental to your body as the 1929 stock market fiasco was to the worldwide economy. Normally, when your blood sugar drops below a critical level, affecting your thinking ability as well as your general health (you may feel light-headed, weak, anxious, and sick to your stomach), your body calls on glucagon.

Glucagon is a hormone. It works with insulin to regulate your blood sugar levels. In fact, glucagon is insulin's foil. As you've heard, insulin moves glucose out of your bloodstream into your body cells. Glucagon does the opposite. This hormone activates the breakdown of glycogen, causing blood sugar levels to rise.

> ### SIT UP STRAIGHT
>
> Crystal-clear thinking can be as easy as straightening yourself out, literally.
>
> Research shows that good posture not only projects health and confidence while hunching says "I'm weak," but it also increases blood flow to your brain. Your brain thrives on a constant source of glucose, sometimes called "blood sugar."
>
> When you let your body sag, two arteries passing through the spinal column may get squeezed, causing an inadequate blood supply. The result? Poor thinking.
>
> So straighten yourself out. Keep your shoulders squared and your head erect. Poor posture is a hard habit to break, but the brainy benefits are worth the effort.

However, after pigging out on sugar and experiencing the crash, your insulin level still remains high for hours. Some researchers believe that the brain, tricked into thinking it has ample glucose, may not enlist glucagon's help.

So your brain—in need of a glucose fix, pronto—may send an S.O.S. for more sugar. You get a craving for sweets and usually give in. Your brain is happy again, but not for long. When blood sugar levels plummet again, it tunes out.

And I bet you thought your "must eat chocolate" mantra signaled a lack of willpower. To the contrary, fulfilling food cravings has everything to do with your biochemistry. (More on cravings in chapter 4).

The trick to avoiding the vicious cycle of high and low blood sugar is staying away from sugary foods and drinks. Does this mean you ought never to eat sweets? No. Just remember that eating them may cause brain drain, so save your sweet snacks for times that you don't need to think well, and eat them in small amounts along with complex carbohydrates and protein to blunt sugar's effect on your insulin level.

▪ An Ironclad Brain ▪

While you dine on healthy amounts of fat and sugar, don't skimp on iron, for a smart reason: Research shows that getting enough iron boosts brain power.

Before I looked at the latest studies, I thought the case on iron was overstated and made little sense. Get this: The Recommended Dietary Allowance (RDA) is 15 milligrams for women in their child-bearing years, an amount that's difficult to take in through foods, and the RDA for pregnant women is twice that amount. (Men need only 10 milligrams of iron daily.) Then, a few years ago, well-respected studies found that men and women who have high iron stores may be at increased risk for heart disease.

Now I have a new respect for this mineral. Yet I do not go out of my way to eat a ton of it. And I've been a vegetarian for more than a dozen years. Here's why.

As you may know, some dietitians think many vegetarians and almost vegetarians don't get enough iron. Meat contains heme iron, a form that the body absorbs more easily than nonheme iron. About 60 percent of the iron in meat and all of the iron in plant foods, eggs, and dairy products is in this more poorly absorbed form. In fact, the body absorbs 2 to 20 percent of nonheme iron, compared to 15 to 35 percent of heme iron.

The variability in the absorption rates depends on you: The lower your iron stores, the more your body absorbs from food, research shows. Some foods—like tea, legumes, and whole grains—can interfere with iron absorption, while other foods help it along. A perfect example is vitamin C. When you eat an orange or drink six ounces of citrus juice with a meal, your absorption of nonheme iron may double.

Curiously, though meat has abundant iron, surveys indicate that vegetarians consume more iron than people who eat meat regularly. Yet the prevailing belief about iron and vegetarians is that they're at increased risk of developing iron-deficiency anemia. The research, while admittedly not extensive, tells a different story.

For instance, in a controlled study by the U.S. Department of Agriculture, researchers compared the blood iron levels of a group of women—half of whom dined on six ounces of meat daily while the other half ate a vegetarian diet including eggs and cheese. When the researchers measured the women's iron stores after seven weeks, they found equivalent levels in both groups.

Now for the bad news: Iron deficiency is the most common nutrient deficiency in the United States. In fact, one in five women of childbearing age is iron deficient. Low iron stores can affect your energy, cognitive function, even your IQ.

Fortunately, the Power-Up Food Plan provides a healthy dose of iron. To take no chances, talk to your doctor or other health practitioner about getting a serum ferritin test, which measures your iron stores. If your stores are low, consider supplementation. If they're fine, relax.

Clearly, your brain needs iron. Research shows that children and adults who eat an iron-poor diet are more likely to have learning disabilities. Too little iron in the diet can also lead to

---

WHAT ABOUT WHITE BREAD?

One prominent nutrition researcher had said that refined carbohydrates like white bread and pasta should be lumped together with sugar, an empty calorie food.

Why? Refined carbos, even if they aren't sugary like cupcakes, are digested more quickly than unrefined carbos like whole-wheat bread, brown rice, legumes, vegetables, and fruits. This means that to regulate blood sugar levels, the body may release the hormone insulin at a hurried pace, setting off the highs and lows of the sugar boogie blues.

But hold on to your bagels.

Though refined carbos lack many of the nutrients and most of the fiber found in unrefined carbos, they're still carbos and not sugar. Enzymes must break down their chains of glucose molecules into single molecules.

In addition, most meals that include refined carbos also contain fiber-rich foods. An example is pasta with chunky tomato sauce, a salad, and garlic bread. Though the pasta and garlic bread are refined carbos, the vegetables in the sauce and salad are not. The latter have fiber, which slows digestion.

And your favorite bagel? Eat it with some cream cheese and a piece of fruit. The fat in the cream cheese and the fiber in the fruit also slow digestion.

The point is, pair refined carbos with healthier unrefined foods, and you'll still enjoy the benefits of power-eating.

lowered intelligence, poor concentration, shortened attention span, lack of motivation, and suboptimal performance in school and at work.

Why does brain function nose-dive when your iron is low?

First, your brain suffocates. Because iron is essential for transporting oxygen to your brain, your brain is starved for air when your iron is low.

Second, without adequate oxygen, your cells

> **5 WAYS TO AVOID THE AFTERNOON SLUMP**
>
> *Do* eat lunch. Skipping your midday meal robs your brain of its fuel—glucose.
>
> *Don't* eat big. Energy is diverted to your stomach for digestion, so the more you eat, the less energy you'll have for clear thinking.
>
> *Do* choose primarily whole grains, vegetables, and fruit, which digest gradually.
>
> *Don't* eat only carbos at lunch. Have some protein-rich legumes, low-fat cheese, or yogurt to keep you mentally agile.
>
> *Do* take a walk, climb stairs, rollerblade, or lift weights at midday. By moving, your body pumps more blood and gets extra fuel to your brain.

cannot convert glucose into energy to meet your needs. As a result, you feel tired and cannot think clearly or quickly.

A case in point: Researchers at Johns Hopkins School of Medicine in Baltimore screened 716 Baltimore high school girls and found eighty-one who were iron deficient but not severely enough to cause anemia. Each girl received either 260 milligrams of iron or a look-alike placebo twice a day. After eight weeks, the girls who took iron scored better on a test of verbal learning and memory than did the girls who got the placebo.

Remember, the only way to be sure your iron supply is adequate (and brain empowering) is to get tested. Reversing iron deficiency is quite easy. Eat iron-rich foods, like legumes, spinach, dried apricots, raisins, and lima beans, and maximize iron absorption by eating a vitamin C–rich food along with an iron-rich food. Another trick: Cook some of your meals in cast-iron pots.

■ REMEMBER WHEAT GERM? ■

Wheat germ, eggs, and soybeans have something in common: choline, the key to better memory and overall brain function. It may also figure in to the prevention of age-related memory loss, seen in Alzheimer's victims, for example.

Choline is a B vitamin–like substance that's the building block of acetylcholine, the memory manager neurotransmitter. When your acetylcholine levels are low, you cannot easily store or retrieve information. Not surprisingly, in studies in which people were given a drug that blocks acetylcholine, they flunked memory tests, but scored super high when given a drug that increases acetylcholine levels.

The best news: The more choline you eat, the more gets to your brain.

That means improving your memory is as close as a jar of wheat germ. Wheat germ, eggs, and soybeans (and soybeans' cousins, including tofu, tempeh, and soymilk) are the richest nutritional sources of choline. It's also found in lecithin, a supplement you can find in natural food stores and pharmacies. Store-bought lecithin may contain as little as 30 percent choline, so its potency remains questionable.

Some researchers believe that long-term choline deficiency may be at the root of Alzheimer's disease. While it's unclear

---

A BRAINY BREAKFAST

You've heard it before: The smart way to start your day is by eating a good breakfast.

Countless studies have shown that people perform better on memory and attention tests and get better grades in school or on the job when they eat breakfast. Eating breakfast boosts your blood-glucose level, which dwindles during a night of sleep. The boost in blood glucose translates to greater brain power.

So, is the ideal breakfast platefuls of pancakes, eggs, hash browns, juice, and milk? No.

The smartest breakfast has a moderate amount of calories (about 500), is low in fat and high in carbohydrates, is vitamin-rich, and includes a protein food.

Hmmm. It seems to me that a big bowl of raisin brain with skim milk is just right. And so is oatmeal with soymilk and a glass of orange juice. Or yogurt with chopped fruit and granola. Or scrambled eggs with toast and fruit. Or . . . the possibilities are deliciously countless.

whether this disease can be reversed by increasing choline in the diet, studies have shown that it can be slowed.

But why wait? Increasing your choline intake, which automatically raises acetylcholine levels in your brain, powers up your brain now. Remember when you tried to identify what's-her-name? Eat choline, and you probably will.

Fill up on antioxidants too. They protect your brain

> **SMART SNACKS**
>
> An oversized low-fat bran muffin
> A fruit smoothie
> Plain nonfat yogurt with cut-up fruit stirred in
> Low-fat cottage cheese with a sprinkle of cinnamon
> A small handful of Brazil nuts
> A bagel topped with fruit chutney
> Pita bread stuffed with lettuce, tomato, bell pepper, and low-fat creamy dressing
> Baked tortilla chips and salsa
> A soft pretzel
> A bowl of air-popped popcorn with a smidgeon of melted butter
>
>

by preventing damage to cells crucial to thinking smart. More on antioxidants in chapter 6.

■ THE SMART NUTRIENTS ■

Optimal brain power depends on a slew of nutrients. If you're deficient in any single one of them, you may not think as well as you could.

For instance, a study showed that thiamin-deficient children who later supplemented their diet with this vitamin scored better on intelligence and memory tests after one year. Another study found that men aged seventy to seventy-nine years who took in extra B_6 (found in such foods as green peas, bananas, leafy greens, and brown rice) had a better long-term memory and an improved capacity to store information in the brain compared to age-matched men who did not supplement their diets with B_6.

Still another study found that mild nutritional deficits in thiamin in twenty-eight people aged sixty years and older changed brain waves and impaired cognitive performance. Similarly, skimping on boron, a trace mineral in nuts and fruits, may impair your brain. In one research study, fifteen people over age forty-five ate little boron over four months, and their brains produced more theta waves and fewer alpha waves, causing a mental slowdown. When their intake of boron was increased, their brain wave activity picked up too.

As mentioned, the Recommended Dietary Allowances (RDAs), considered the standard for assessing nutritional status, are based on the physical symptoms of nutritional deficiencies. But long before physical symptoms appear, the brain shows changes in thinking, memory, and intelligence—for the worse. You may notice that you're less sharp mentally (i.e., you no longer win at Scrabble), but probably blame stress, bad luck, or older age.

The truth is, you can stay smart or, if necessary, reclaim your brain power. Along with eating protein-rich foods at the right times, cutting down on fat and sugar, getting a healthy amount of iron, and increasing your intake of choline, fork in the smart nutrients.

Here, in alphabetical order, are the most important ones and their best food sources:

Biotin: Soy foods, peanut butter, whole grains, and dairy products.

Boron: Soy foods, prunes, raisins, peanuts, and hazelnuts.

B vitamins: Bran, wheat germ, legumes, whole grains, nuts, soy foods, dairy products, eggs, broccoli, bananas, carrots, leafy greens, oranges, and fortified cereal.

Iron: Legumes, bran, whole grains, leafy greens, prunes, raisins, dried apricots, and lima beans.

Zinc: Bran, eggs, soy foods, wheat germ, whole grains, and blackstrap molasses.

■ COFFEE, TEA, OR . . . CHOCOLATE ■

Nearly a decade ago, when I worked at *Vegetarian Times,* two of the assignment editors had a ritual I could set my clock by. Every afternoon at the same time, they headed down Lake Street to a gourmet coffee shop and ordered cappuccinos. They got a caffeine boost that fueled the afternoon's work of assigning stories and rewriting, tasks that require intense concentration and mental creativity.

Back then, I looked down on caffeine as a drug—a legal one, but still a drug—and didn't appreciate its power as a brain pick-me-up. So it surprised me to discover numerous studies showing that low doses of caffeine can improve mental performance.

In one experiment, for instance, the participants took various doses of caffeine, ranging from 32 milligrams in soda pop to 256 milligrams in a ten-ounce mug of brewed coffee. All the participants, even those taking the smallest doses, improved their performance on mental tests measuring concentration, reaction time, attention span, and accuracy with numbers.

Caffeine loading (drinking several cups of coffee, tea, or soda) doesn't provide extra brain power. In fact, caffeine loading usually backfires; it can make you jittery and impair clear thinking.

The best dose: 100 to 200 milligrams a day.

The best timing: Half shortly upon awakening and half with your midday meal. A shot of caffeine at midday can counteract the common post-lunch dip in mental performance by increasing alertness.

The biggest no-no: Drinking coffee or tea if you're sensitive to the effects of caffeine, as I am. The easiest way to tell is by observing how you feel about a half hour after taking in a moderate amount. Are you anxious? jittery? tense? agitated? If you answer yes, you're probably sensitive to caffeine. Avoid it altogether or have it in tiny amounts.

Like in a chocolate kiss.

A single kiss has only a couple of milligrams of caffeine. It also contains theobromine, a substance similar to caffeine. Theobromine increases alertness, concentration, and overall mental functioning, too.

Karin and Debra can keep their cappuccinos. I'm choosing chocolate.

▪ THE BRAIN-POWER CUSTOMIZER ▪

Here's the first of several Customizers that show you how to eat for your specific needs. This one pays special attention to your thinking abilities, including concentration, memory, creativity, and general mental aptitude. Follow the Power-Up Food Plan (chapter 7) and emphasize the following:

1. Eat brain-power foods and avoid brain-drain foods.

BRAIN-POWER FOODS	BRAIN-DRAIN FOODS

Lean protein
    Legumes, including soy foods,
    low-fat dairy products,
    high-protein grains,
    egg whites (with an occasional
        yolk)
	Fatty protein
	    Steak, lunchmeat,
	    full-fat dairy
	    products

Nutrient-rich
    Bran, wheat germ, whole
    grains, nuts (in moderation),
    oranges, bananas, dried apricots,
    raisins, prunes, leafy greens
	Nutrient-poor
	    Butter, margarine,
	    chips, cookies,
	    cake, pie, candy

Low-sugar
    Fruit, unsweetened fruit spread,
    unsweetened applesauce,
    seltzer water
	High-sugar
	    Fruited yogurt, candy,
	    most baked goods, ice
	    cream, frozen yogurt

Other
    100 to 200 milligrams
    of caffeine a day
	Other
	    More than 200
	    milligrams of caffeine a day

2. Eat brain-power foods at the right times.

To start your day with mental energy, eat a lean protein at breakfast. Smart picks: corn flakes with skim milk or low-fat soymilk, low-fat yogurt with fruit, or a low-fat cheese-and-vegetable omelet. Dumb picks: toast or blintzes with fruit juice but no protein food (such as milk or soy-based sausages).

Eat a lean protein at lunch to avoid an afternoon slump in energy and alertness. Smart picks: bean burritos, black bean soup with breadsticks, a soy-based burger, or a low-fat cheese-and-vegetable sandwich. Dumb picks: a vegetable or fruit salad with rolls, or a vegetable sauté with rice but no protein food (such as legumes or tofu).

To keep up brain power, eat a lean protein at dinner too. Smart picks: cheese ravioli, spinach and mushroom calzone, or a frittata. Dumb picks: pasta with marinara sauce, or vegetable kebabs with couscous but no protein food.

For snacks, include a lean protein. Smart picks: bean dip and baked tortilla chips, or low-fat cheese and crackers. Dumb picks: ice cream, cookies, or potato chips.

An exception: When you need brain power but you feel anxious, tense, nervous, or jittery, eat a small carbo-only snack. Eaten without protein, the snack will kick

---

THINGS WORTH AVOIDING

While boosting brain power, do nothing to risk it. Here are five common brain-drains you should try to avoid.

1. Lead. This toxic metal can reduce IQ and cause brain damage when ingested or inhaled. Americans today average 500 times more lead in their bodies than people in preindustrial times.
Smart moves:

- Don't eat on china that contains lead. Most likely culprits are colored and imported types. To be certain, ask the manufacturer.
- Don't use any cleaning products that contain lead.
- Safely remove any lead paint from your home.
- Replace plumbing that has lead solders.

2. Pesticides. Eating foods laced with pesticides may contribute to disease, including dementia. Among the worst offenders are some crops imported by other countries where chemicals banned in the United States are legal to use.
Smart moves:

- Buy certified organic produce, which by definition has been grown without pesticides.
- Wash your produce. A thorough cleaning will remove most pesticide residues.
- Grow a garden. Then you have complete control and full knowledge of how the foods have been treated.

3. Smoke. Did you know that smoking reduces oxygen supply to the brain, causing impaired mental function?
Smart moves:

- Always request seating in the nonsmoking section of a restaurant. Secondhand smoke is dangerous too.

- If you still smoke, please try quitting again. Studies suggest that smokers usually make several attempts before they're successful.

4. Alcohol. Drinking too much alcohol too often can damage your nerves, leading to memory loss, poor concentration, and even personality changes.

Smart moves:

- If you drink, do so in moderation. That means no more than one drink daily for women and two drinks daily for men.
- Never drink until you're drunk.
- If you suspect that you or a loved one might have a drinking problem, seek help.

5. Stress. Stress not only monkeys with your moods but also with brain power. People with chronic or acute stress may have poor memory and concentration. High blood pressure, which often accompanies excessive stress, is linked to shortened attention span too.

Smart moves:

- Learn to say no. When you turn down an offer to chair the PTA or to take on an extra work project, you have time for yourself.
- Pay attention to physical signs of stress. Headaches, backaches, and intestinal distress may signal stress months before it shows up as anxiety, irritability, or depression.
- Take a break. As stress increases, you may need to decrease your activities. That may mean taking a sabbatical from work, resigning your post as your daughter's Girl Scout troop leader, hiring help to clean your house or mow the lawn, or anything else your innate wisdom suggests that you do.

in serotonin, the neurotransmitter that calms nerves and helps you think better when you're keyed up. If possible, time the snack for thirty minutes prior to your need for a brain boost.

3. Eat brain-power foods in the right combos.

- A protein food with or without carbos.
- A protein food with nutrient-rich foods.
- Iron-rich foods (such as legumes or spinach) with a vitamin C food to boost iron absorption.

Brain-power tip of the day: When you need to think well, eat a lean protein with or without carbos, but never eat carbos alone (unless you're feeling anxious).

POWER QUIZ

Brain Boost or Brain Drain?

Are you as smart as you think you are? smarter? Your yes or no answers will reveal how well you're taking care of your brain and reaping smart benefits.

1. Do you sleep at least seven hours a night?
   _____ yes _____ no

2. Do you avoid large meals, especially at lunch?
   _____ yes _____ no

3. Do you only rarely eat full-size sugary treats like candy bars or ice cream? _____ yes _____ no

4. Do you occasionally allow yourself small sugary treats?
   _____ yes _____ no

5. Do you take some time for yourself each day—a walk, a bath, or some other relaxing activity?
   _____ yes _____ no

6. Do you engage in regular aerobic exercise, like swimming or dance? _____ yes _____ no

7. Do you eat foods rich in the following nutrients every day?
   Vitamin C: _____ yes _____ no
   Vitamin E: _____ yes _____ no
   Beta-carotene: _____ yes _____ no
   Selenium: _____ yes _____ no

8. Do you limit your alcohol consumption to no more than one drink a day? _____ yes _____ no

9. Do you often avoid foods with more than 3 grams of fat per serving? _____ yes _____ no

10. Do you limit your intake of saturated fat?
    _____ yes _____ no

11. Do you limit your intake of trans fatty acids (most easily identified on product ingredient lists as "hydrogenated" or "partially hydrogenated")?

_____ yes _____ no

12. When you use oil, do you typically choose olive or canola oil? _____ yes _____ no

13. Do you avoid crash diets? _____ yes _____ no

14. Do you always eat breakfast?

_____ yes _____ no

15. Do you typically eat five or more meals or snacks each day?

_____ yes _____ no

16. If you're a woman, do you typically eat at least 2,000 calories daily? If you're a man, do you typically eat at least 2,500 calories daily? _____ yes _____ no

17. Do you eat eggs, wheat germ, or soy foods a few times a week?

_____ yes _____ no

18. Do you get ample dietary fiber from whole grains, vegetables, fruits, and legumes? _____ yes _____ no

19. Do you rarely feel mentally fuzzy?

_____ yes _____ no

20. Do you rarely forget where you've placed your things?

_____ yes _____ no

21. Would you describe yourself as usually alert and mentally agile, with little difficulty concentrating on the task at hand?

_____ yes _____ no

_____

Now give yourself a point for each yes answer and tally your score. The highest possible score is 24.

If you scored 20 to 24 points, you're in the brainy bunch.

Did you score 15 to 19 points? You have moments of brain power and of brain drain.

A score lower than 15 points means you can substantially improve your brain power and reap the benefits: improved concentration, greater alertness, better memory and creativity, and quicker and clearer thinking. What are you waiting for?

## three

Good-bye, Blues!
Hello, Mood Power!

The ingredients of a good mood are simple: energy and calm. These are turned on and off by many things, most particularly your food choices and stress levels, with the help of—you guessed it—your neurotransmitters.

These biochemical messengers, which pass important chunks of information among your neurons (brain cells), "tell" you to feel lethargic and run-down, or vigorous and energized; anxious and stressed out, or calm and content. The calmer and more energetic you feel, the greater your mood power.

Before we look at how to rev up and calm down—and, later in the chapter, how to say so long to PMS and the blues—let's consider Mary and her mood, food choices, and stress. You'll get a picture of how the three intertwine.

Eleven A.M. Mary, a thirty-year-old executive secretary, is working at her desk. Four hours earlier, she power-ate a breakfast of high-fiber, fortified cereal with skim milk and fruit. So now she's relaxed and focuses easily on her work.

If you asked her how she feels, she might describe her mood as upbeat, energetic, calm, and happy. Robert E. Thayer, Ph.D., author of *The Origin of Everyday Moods,* calls it *calm-energy,* one of four basic moods he describes in his book. It's the optimal mood, the state we'd consistently describe in glowing terms.

One P.M. Mary's stomach is rumbling as she heads out for

lunch. Unexpectedly, one of her three managers stops her and gives her a project with a three o'clock deadline. She senses that her job performance rating will go up if she does well.

So Mary grabs the box of crackers she keeps in her desk and munches on them as she scans her new project. She swivels her chair to face her computer screen, and her fingers fly to make the dozen graphics her manager needs. Meanwhile, in her brain, her walnut-sized hypothalamus is signaling the release of stress hormones, increasing her heart rate and metabolism. Her shoulder and neck muscles tighten.

She is trying to concentrate on her work, but her eyes dart frequently to the clock. Her thoughts are somewhat scattered, which unnerves her a bit, because she needs to focus.

This is *tense-energy*. A psychologist might diagnose low-level anxiety, but she'd probably say she feels fairly good. Mary, like others I know, thrives in the tense-energy state, as long as it doesn't overstay its welcome. When it drags on, nervousness and irritability rear up.

Five P.M. Mary fights rush-hour traffic on the way home, but has enough energy to create a simple meal of pasta topped with marinara sauce and a romaine salad. After dinner, she strolls around the neighborhood for some exercise and relaxation. Back home, she curls up on the recliner and watches a videotape of her favorite soap opera.

Her body has shifted into low drive. Her energy reserves are nearly tapped out, but she's content. This is *calm-tiredness,* a generally pleasant mood.

Seven A.M the next morning. Having tossed and turned through the night, Mary is tired and late for work. She grabs a bagel and gobbles it in the car. At the office, she works feverishly into the afternoon, when she finally breaks for a pitiful lunch of frozen yogurt and a banana. She feels worn out.

Six P.M. Mary goes straight home, fighting traffic in pouring rain, which causes her to feel more worn out and uptight, and she skips her aerobics class. Throwing in the towel on exercise is quite common for a person who, like Mary, is in the state of *tense-tiredness.* If you ask her how she feels, her one-word answer ought to be clear: "Bad!"

When tense-tired, our bodies sense a "danger" and our minds go nuts trying to locate it. We're stuck in a bad mood, unless we think our way out of it (hard—just try it) or we eat, exercise, and relax our way to contentment (much easier, much more satisfying). Check out chapters 8 and 9, for details on power-cising and power-living, respectively.

To recap, the four main moods are:

calm-energy, the optimal state
tense-energy
calm-tiredness
tense-tiredness, which can underlie depression

There is a fifth mood state: exhaustion. Exhaustion occurs when your resources are depleted. Even with tense-tiredness, you still can get going and accomplish some tasks, though you may feel like plopping in front of the TV (a distraction technique) or have a compulsion to ruminate on your problems, real or perceived, hoping to figure out why you feel so darn lousy.

Fortunately, research suggests an escape hatch to mood power: the right foods—carbos for calm, protein for energy, and a wee bit of fat for a perk.

■ CARBOS FOR CALM ■

Carbohydrates, or carbos for short, are a launching pad to food-induced serenity. Whether you eat complex carbohydrates (whole grains, legumes, vegetables) or simple carbohydrates (soda pop, candy, sweet baked goods), these pick-me-ups can enhance your mood by pushing your biochemical button for serotonin.

As mentioned, serotonin, the "comforting" neurotransmitter, helps regulate mood as well as sleep, food intake, and pain tolerance. When your brain levels of serotonin are adequate, you feel your very best. When they're low, you may become depressed, anxious, or lethargic or experience a similar downer emotion. The severity depends on how low your serotonin levels have dropped, your genetic weakness for bad mood, your diet, and other factors.

Remember that your serotonin levels are directly related to your diet, particularly to the carbo content of your latest meal or snack:

bad mood (anxiety, depression, and so on) → eat carbos only → brain levels of tryptophan increase → serotonin levels increase → improved mood

or

> HYPOGLYCEMIA: IS IT FOR REAL?
>
> In a word, yes.
>
> Hypoglycemia, or low blood sugar, is a condition, not a disease. Between meals, blood sugar levels drop to between 60 and 110 milligrams per deciliter. When they go below 40 milligrams per deciliter, you experience hypoglycemia and its symptoms: rapid heartbeat, trembling, sweating, and hunger.
>
> In reactive hypoglycemia, the body dumps a load of the hormone insulin into your bloodstream, causing blood sugar to drop well below normal, after a large or sugar-filled meal. The symptoms mentioned above may occur, but not until two to four hours after the meal.
>
> Though hypoglycemia is a bona fide medical condition, the jury is out on its prevalence, with some docs believing it's rare and other docs saying it's fairly common.
>
> If you suspect hypoglycemia, talk to your doctor or health practitioner about testing your blood glucose level while you're experiencing symptoms for a clear diagnosis. Meanwhile, avoid sugary meals and snacks and at the first sign of symptoms eat a nutritious snack like fruit, which digests quickly and raises blood sugar levels.

bad mood (anxiety, depression, and so on) → eat protein or a carbo-protein mix → brain levels of tryptophan stagnate → serotonin levels do not rise → continuation of bad mood

■ PROTEIN FOR ENERGY ■

When you're calm yet hunger for energy—and, remember, energy is a main component of good mood—eat protein. Protein itself doesn't fuel your energy tanks. Carbos do. Rather, eating protein stops the amino acid tryptophan from entering your brain. No tryptophan, no serotonin.

When you eat a protein food like milk (dairy or soy), low-fat yogurt or cheese, or a soy-based burger, your energy level will increase and you'll feel perky and happier.

But isn't serotonin, you ask, the super-mood neurotransmitter?

Yes. So please do go for the carbo gusto when you're anxious, tense, jittery, depressed, or the like.

But if you eat a carbo-only meal or snack when you're already calm and content, the rise in serotonin will probably curtail your energy and damper your mood. That's because the amino acid tyrosine (not to be confused with tryptophan) cannot get to your brain and make the "alertness" neurotransmitters dopamine and norepinephrine.

low energy → eat protein or a carbo-protein mix → brain levels of tyrosine increase → serotonin is not manufactured while dopamine and norepinephrine rise → greater energy

Underscoring the importance of protein for energy and mood is a study by researchers at the United States Army Research Institute of Environmental Medicine in Massachusetts. They tested the effects of tyrosine supplements on soldiers in progressively harsher and more stressful conditions.

At the most extreme, the test conditions simulated being lifted suddenly to an elevation of 15,500 feet, causing a drop in oxygen available to the brain, and being exposed, in lightweight clothing, to 60 degrees Fahrenheit.

Tests showed that the soldiers who had taken tyrosine supplements not only reported better moods but also had superior mental energy to perform such tasks as charting coordinates on a map, translating messages into code, and making complex decisions.

Just remember: for energy eat protein, but for greater calm go for the carbos.

Or fat.

■ FAT FOR A PERK ■

Wonderfully, some research, while still far from conclusive, is showing that eating a small amount of fat—as in two or three chocolate kisses—may help cause the release of endorphins, which I've nicknamed the "ooh-la-la" neurotransmitter.

With low endorphin levels, you may feel fatigued and stressed out (the combo for a bad mood) and your body may scream, "Give me a fat now!" If you don't fulfill your desire, you'll still feel crummy. But when you listen—that's a story with a happy ending.

low endorphins → bad mood (tired and tense) → desire for fat → eat fatty foods → increase in endorphins → pleasurable mood

---

HIGH-ENERGY FOOD TIPS

Don't accept fatigue lying down. You can fight back and reenergize yourself quickly and painlessly. Here are top picks.

- Enjoy a satisfying breakfast of complex carbos, some protein, and little fat if desired—every day.
- Eat frequently (three meals plus two or three snacks daily) to maintain a healthy blood sugar level. Your brain thrives on a steady flow of glucose.
- Go for carbos only when you're anxious, uptight, nervous, or tense. Anxiety can zap your energy. Otherwise, eat a mix of carbos and protein.
- Get enough nutrients, particularly iron, the B vitamins, and magnesium. Suboptimal levels of these nutrients may make you as slow as a slug.
- Spare the fat. A fat-heavy meal diverts blood away from your brain. The result: a severe lack of energy.
- Only one lump, please. When you shovel in sugar, your body does the sugar boogie: you go up, then down, eat some more sugar, go up, down, eat more sugar, up, down. You get the idea. So eat sugary foods infrequently and reach for satisfying complex carbos like whole-wheat bread, apples, and corn.
- Have a cup or two of java a day, and no more. If you're a coffee, tea, or cola drinker, the caffeine in your brew gives you an energy lift as long as you don't take in too much. But when you drink more than two cups a day, you may feel uptight and jittery—and de-energized.

Says my friend Rema: "I eat chocolate when I'm feeling run-down or low emotionally. After I eat it, I feel perked up. I feel soothed. I don't have to have a lot of chocolate, but when I need it, I really need it."

▪ A MOOD BUSTER ▪

Our faster-is-better culture deplores idleness and leaves us little time to stop and smell the roses. The sad truth is, many of us are no longer human *beings* but human *doers*. Overworked, time-crunched, I-need-a-vacation-now! human doers. Our busyness often leads to stress, and stress sets up fatigue (the opposite of energy) and anxiety (the opposite of calm).

excessive stress → reduced energy and increased anxiety → bad mood

Juliet R. Schor, author of *The Overworked American: The Unexpected Decline of Leisure* and a Harvard University economist, says our work time has been increasing since 1960 and that the average American owns and consumes twice as much today as his or her counterpart did some forty years ago. In contrast,

- A Roman living in the fourth century enjoyed 200 holidays a year; a medieval peasant had 115.
- Today's Europeans, after a year of employment, average five or six weeks of paid vacation a year. Americans usually get only two weeks.

As mentioned, whether your stress is physical or emotional, your body reacts with a series of biochemical changes. It releases various stress hormones that jump-start your body. Your pupils dilate, muscles tense, reflexes sharpen, the heartbeat quickens. When stress is continual, your body has trouble handling the load of stress hormones.

One way that your body tries to protect itself against excessive stress is by turning on your craving for carbos. It releases neuropeptide Y (NPY), the appetite-stimulating neurotransmitter. Remember, carbos calm you. When you eat them without protein, your body makes "comforting" serotonin.

stress → release of cortisol and other stress hormones → increase of NPY → desire for carbos → eat carbos → increase of serotonin → improved mood

I'm sure you have your burnout story. I've certainly got mine.

I was fresh out of college and had landed a job with a daily newspaper as a reporter on the late-night crime beat. When the police scanner was quiet, I was as bored as an eight-year-old on a rainy day with nothing to do. But when the police dispatcher sent fire trucks to a blazing house with people trapped inside or squad cars to a robbery in progress or a coroner to a murder scene, I summoned a photographer and grabbed the car keys. As we raced toward the disaster, I was on an incredible adrenaline high.

Seeing my byline on page one the next day gave me a momentary lift. Yet over the months the continual stress attacked my weak spot. Yours may be a propensity toward headaches or digestive problems. Mine is the jitters.

My diet suffered too. Although I ate fairly nutritious breakfasts and lunches, my dinners were fast-food burgers and fries. (This was before my vegetarian days.) At work, I drank can after can of caffeinated diet soda pop and dropped pocketfuls of change into the vending machine for bags of peanut M&Ms.

I needed my fix. That's right: Through food, I medicated myself, seeking a mood boost from caffeine and a serotonin lift from sugar. My brain desired calm-energy, but between my job stress, bad food choices, and creeping anxiety (and extra pounds, which made me feel worse inside and out), I set myself up for tense-tiredness. Fortunately, I quit my job as a crime reporter before I ended up in a psych ward.

Stress plays other tricks. It steps up your metabolic rate, causing nutrients (and neurotransmitters) to be burned up quickly. When under severe stress, you also need extra calories, protein, and carbohydrates. Stress weakens your immune system too.

While feeling low now and then is only human, unrelenting fatigue and anxiety spell trouble. Be sure to consult your doctor or health practitioner if a bad mood sticks to you like Velcro.

So how can the stressed-out say au revoir to bad moods?

First, realize that you are experiencing moderate-to-high levels of stress and decide that you must get off the treadmill to feel good again. Second, make healthy lifestyle choices, including exercising, having quiet time, and enjoying hobbies. Third, power-eat.

Remember, stress begets anxiety begets poor food choices. That's what happened to me fifteen years ago when I made bad food choices and shoveled in junk—sugar, fat, caffeine, and meat. Though it can be tough to eat powerfully under stress of any kind—a messy divorce, the death of a loved one, even relocating for your dream job—don't make the mistake I did.

Promise to yourself that you'll choose serene cuisine. The feel-good payoff is worth it.

▪ THE GOOD-MOOD CUSTOMIZER ▪

You need carbos *and* protein—and a little fat too—to power your mood. You just need to know what, when, and how. Follow the Power-Up Food Plan (chapter 7) and emphasize the following:

1. Eat good-mood foods.

To ward off anxiety, depression, the jitters, tenseness, irritability, and other downer feelings: carbos.

For greater energy when you're already calm: protein.

To lift your spirits: a smidgeon of fat, especially chocolate.

Here are some examples:

CALM-DOWN CARBOS	ENERGETIC PROTEIN	BIG-LIFT FATS
Bruschetta	Quiche	Chocolate
Whole-grain bagel	Veggie burger	Peanut butter cookie
Mashed potatoes	Bean burrito	Ice cream
Angel hair pasta	Lentil soup	Cupcake
Blueberry muffin	Cheese omelette	Brownie
Herbed focaccia	Hummus	Baked Alaska

2. Eat good-mood foods at the right times.

Carbos anytime you are tense or depressed, especially early in the morning and late in the evening (and in the late afternoon, too, if you have energy).

A carbo-protein mix throughout the day, unless you feel tense or tired—then eat a carbo meal or snack.

Fat in moderation for a pick-me-up.

3. Eat good-mood foods in the right combos.

Carbos alone when tense.

When you feel energetic and calm, a carbo-protein mix at meals and snacks, or protein alone (example: a glass of skim milk as a snack).

Fat alone or, even better, in a creamy-sweet combo like ice cream.

■ SO LONG, PMS ■

Swayed by the "embrace thyself" mantra of the likes of mind-body guru Deepak Chopra, the popular women's magazines are making a woman's menstrual cycle sound like a stroll through a rose garden in bloom. "Celebrate," they chant, and "Appreciate the power of your femininity." And lest I forget: "Honor your reproductive cycles, which wax and wane with the moon, giving you a special bond to Mother Nature."

These saccharine proclamations curl my cuticles, I confess. Most women would rather forget about our uniquely female experience. But truly there is reason for joy.

Women are life-givers. Our fertility cycles give opportunity for conception and birth and relationships, not only with our mates but also with our children, other women, and our communities. Nowadays it's not uncommon for a mother to give her daughter a special gift to mark her becoming a woman, signaled by menarche.

But wait a sec.

This is sounding too schmaltzy and surreal—or, shall I say, unreal!—to Bonnie, a thirty-something sales rep. The week before her period, she takes on a new persona: Ms. Hyde. She's touchy. She's grouchy. She's ultrasensitive. At the drop of a paper clip, she weeps for no reason—or so it seems.

Bonnie has a nasty case of PMS, an acronym so ingrained in our vernacular that a definition seems unnecessary. For the sake of setting myth-conceptions straight, however, I'll offer one.

PMS, or premenstrual

THE KISS OF CHOCOLATE

If your body tells you to eat chocolate every day, go for it. Chocolate is not some fat fiend poised to make you as round as a bonbon. It's a food you can use to enhance your brain chemistry.

It combines fat and sugar, which some research suggests may boost the endorphins and increase serotonin. Endorphins energize the mind and lift the spirits. Serotonin calms and soothes. As research on mood-enhancing chocolate continues, we'll learn more delicious discoveries about American women's most craved food.

Meanwhile, here's how to enjoy chocolate's luscious kiss now.

Do eat a small amount of chocolate, two chocolate kisses or half of a chocolate bar, whenever you have a biological craving for it.

Don't pig out on a box of the creamy confections. Too much chocolate, which is about one-half fat, will slow digestion and interfere with chocolate's feel-good sensations.

Do fulfill a chocolate craving promptly. If you try to outlast a biological craving, you'll probably get grumpier and may binge.

Don't feel guilty when eating chocolate. Rather, befriend this food. It can be good for you.

Do recognize that eating chocolate has a powerful effect on your brain chemistry. In addition to boosting the endorphins and serotonin levels, it delivers theobromine, a substance similar to caffeine, promoting alertness minus the java jitters, and other substances researchers continue to investigate.

By the way, the legendary lover Casanova proposed that chocolate was better than champagne for romantic interludes. That's the *other* kiss of chocolate.

syndrome, is a catchall for some 150 documented symptoms that occur premenstrually. In other words, PMS occurs during all or part of the fourteen days—give or take a few—between ovulation (when the ovary releases an egg) and the onset of menstruation. PMS symptoms include mood swings, forgetfulness, sadness, anxiety, breast tenderness, bloating, weight gain, headaches, and fatigue. One out of two women in their childbearing years experiences moderate to severe symptoms.

Though some scientific studies have reported no increase of premenstrual tension (i.e., PMS) based on daily self-ratings by women, causing some investigators to infer that PMS may be an excuse for the stress reactions women have, women are convinced it exists. So does the American Psychiatric Association, which includes "late luteal dysphoric disorder" (medical-ese for PMS) in its *Diagnostic and Statistical Manual of Mental Disorders,* the bible of psychiatrists and psychologists.

Yet I submit that PMS is not a disorder. Or a disease. Or a mental disturbance. It's a natural biological event that most women experience during their childbearing years, save for pregnancy. What differs among women is the degree to which we have PMS symptoms.

WHAT CAUSES PMS

Fluctuations in hormones (namely, estrogen and progesterone), prostaglandins (hormonelike substances), and other body chemicals including neurotransmitters bring on PMS symptoms. If your neurotransmitters say, "Feel sad," your emotions will tailspin and you'll feel sad. If they say, "Feel cranky or surly or blah," you will.

But here comes the good news. Though we've come a long way since the days of "the curse," as my grandmother used to call her period, most women needlessly suffer PMS symptoms—until they learn to power-eat. I think of Heidi.

She used to eat the typical American smorgasbord: meat every day, lots of dairy products, some eggs, and white bread, with vegetables and fruit an afterthought. Like most adult Americans who become vegetarian or nearly so, Heidi eliminated animal foods (except fish) to improve her overall health.

Her energy perked up, her weight dropped, and her skin cleared. Another pleasant surprise was no more breast tenderness or moodiness before her period as well as an almost complete disappearance of menstrual cramps. Says Heidi: "Saying so long to PMS was one of the best things that happened to me after I began eating right."

Heidi's story can be yours too. When you power-eat (eating the right foods at the right times in the right combinations), PMS symptoms often lessen or even vanish. Bear with me as I outline a scientific explanation.

During your cycle, two neurotransmitters, the endorphins and serotonin, do a jig that sets you up for the perfect mood, then the worst. That's if you eat the average American diet. When you power-eat, you can boost your feel-good neurotransmitters and counteract PMS symptoms.

Here's how it works.

THE BIOCHEMICAL DANCE

At ovulation, your body makes the endorphins. These neurotransmitters are akin to your own private stash of morphine. And they're free and legal, but "addictive"—in a good way. You'll see what I mean in a moment.

The endorphins help eliminate pain, enhance your creativity, make you feel good, and put you in the mood for sex. It's no accident that your endorphins surge during the forty-eight hours that you are fertile each month. Seemingly obeying by instinct the biblical command to be fruitful and multiply, your body wants to do what you're supposed to do when you're fertile.

After the surge, the endorphins return to normal levels. The problem is, your brain balks during the withdrawal from the high endorphins. This withdrawal during the two weeks before menstruation might make you irritable and emotionally low, and you may have a hankering for high-fat foods.

Picture it this way:

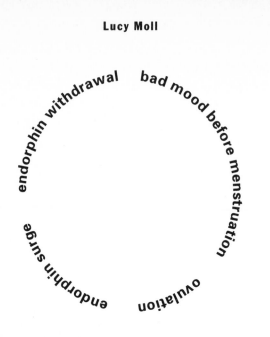

By fulfilling your desire for high-fat foods (in moderation, of course), which, in turn, may boost your endorphin levels, you can ease the endorphin withdrawal. As a result, your mood improves and you're less likely to overeat or choose the wrong foods. Examples of anti-PMS power snacks: a third of a chocolate bar, a big spoonful of ice cream, or even a few tablespoons of safflower oil in a vegetable sauté.

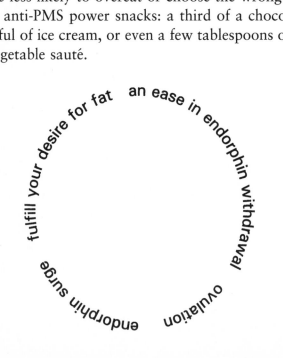

The point is to listen to your body. When your body begs for a creamy treat, feed it. As you learn that nibbling on the right foods makes you feel good, you'll turn to them again and again. The difference between you and a heroin junkie is that you're responding to your biological need for a mood boost with small amounts of *nourishing* food, even if it's chocolate. Never fear: A sweet treat now and then won't undermine your overall good eating habits.

I wish I could honestly report that your body must have a half pound of chocolate or a pint of ultrarich ice cream for you to feel good. But I can't. Some research suggests that at the biochemical level your body needs only a small amount of fat to trigger an endorphin release. If you load up on fat—say, an entire pint of Häagen-Dazs—you're not helping your body, you may feel guilt, and chances are your mood will plunge. More is not better.

low endorphins → bad mood → desire fat → overindulge in fatty foods like ice cream → endorphin release slowed by too much fat → bad mood worsens

Your endorphins are half the story. The "comforting" neurotransmitter serotonin provides the rest.

THE ULTIMATE COMFORT FOOD
Studies confirm that women who feel crummy during the premenstrual phase of their cycle are more likely to eat sweets, with sugar intake increasing to as many as twenty teaspoons daily.

Why sugar?

Simple. As mentioned, eating sugar and other carbohydrates (without protein foods) causes your serotonin levels to waltz like Fred Astaire and Ginger Rogers. This neurotransmitter makes you calm and improves your outlook on life when you're feeling tense or depressed, both of which are common PMS symptoms.

Serotonin levels drop and estrogen and progesterone levels

rise at exactly the same time with the onset of PMS symptoms. As serotonin levels dwindle, you may crave carbos.

> *as estrogen and progesterone levels rise, serotonin levels drop → PMS symptoms, including bad mood → desire for carbos → eat carbos → serotonin levels rise → PMS symptoms decrease*

Hand in hand with a desire for carbos is increased hunger. Food-mood pioneer Judith Wurtman, a nutritional researcher at the Massachusetts Institute of Technology, compared PMS sufferers with women who did not have PMS symptoms and found that on average PMS sufferers increased their daily intake of food from 1,892 calories daily to 2,394 calories daily and their intake of carbos jumped up 24 percent at meals and 43 percent from snacks.

What's clear is PMS sufferers self-medicate with carbos.

To help ease PMS without a carbos binge, Wurtman tested three different drinks on a group of twenty-four women. All three contained carbos but only one was formulated to raise blood levels of the amino acid tryptophan. Neither the women nor the researchers knew who was getting which drink when during the four-month study.

The results: The women who drank the specially formulated concoction felt better. They scored much lower on tests measuring tension, depression, anger, and confusion compared to the women who didn't get the special drink. What's more, the special drink cut their sweet cravings.

When you self-medicate with carbos, do you choose the best anti-PMS foods? Read on to find out.

EATING FOR PMS RELIEF

The best anti-PMS foods are complex carbos like grains and vegetables. When eaten *without* protein foods, complex carbos gradually increase your blood level of the amino acid tryptophan, which floods the brain and triggers the manufacture of serotonin.

Simple carbos like candy, soda pop, and sugary baked goods can also increase your serotonin levels. But there's an unappetizing price you pay. As you've heard, eating simple carbos seats you on a roller coaster ride that costs your mood. (See "The Sugar Boogie Blues" on page 41.)

To counteract PMS symptoms for good:

- Reduce your consumption of saturated fats, which are found primarily in meat and cheese. Research shows that the more animal fats you eat, the higher your blood level of estrogen. Women with estrogen circulating in their blood are more likely to have PMS.
- Eat high-fiber foods like legumes and whole grains. Taking in at least 25 grams of fiber

---

FEELING S.A.D.?

When September breezes in, recharging most of us, the estimated 15 million Americans who suffer seasonal affective disorder, or S.A.D., would rather take a long nap and wake up in April. Shorter days and less sunlight trigger their depression and fatigue. S.A.D. also interferes with sleep and dulls the taste buds.

Often doctors prescribe light treatment (or phototheraphy) to S.A.D. patients. Though the medical community doesn't know exactly why light treatment works, it may suppress overproduction of melatonin, a brain chemical that's key to the body's biological clock.

What you eat can make a difference too. Malatonin is manufactured from serotonin, the "comforting" neurotransmitter. When melatonin levels increase, serotonin levels decrease—and vice versa.

To boost your serotonin levels with food, eat lots of carbos without protein. A carbo-only meal allows the amino acid tryptophan to zip into the brain and make serotonin. In one study, S.A.D. patients who took tryptophan supplements experienced less depression than those given a look-alike capsule.

Ironically, S.A.D. sufferers often are low in the neurotransmitter dopamine. The way to increase your dopamine levels is by eating protein.

So which is best? Carbos or protein?

You'll need to do a little homework to find out what works for you. For one week, log everything you eat and when. Identify whether the meal or snack was carbo-only or high in protein, and gauge your mood before eating and about thirty minutes after.

Then scan your notes and look for patterns. For instance, you might notice that a midafternoon carbo-only snack makes you feel better but carbos in the morning don't. Adjust your eating habits accordingly.

Most important, if you suspect S.A.D., seek medical help. Light therapy appears most effective with the majority of patients. Power-eating along with light therapy might chase away your wintertime blues—at last.

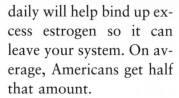

daily will help bind up excess estrogen so it can leave your system. On average, Americans get half that amount.

- Reduce or eliminate your intake of caffeine, which studies have shown may aggravate PMS. Women who drink several cups of caffeinated beverages a day are at greater risk for severe PMS symptoms, including anxiety, depression, breast tenderness, constipation, and acne.
- Choose foods rich in B_6 (and B vitamins in general), vitamin E, iron, magnesium, and calcium, or at the very least consider a nutritional supplement. Studies indicate that a diet poor in these nutrients may worsen PMS symptoms.
- Avoid stress. Stress can aggravate symptoms too. If at all possible, during your premenstrual phase, choose activities that calm you and avoid any extra demands on your time or energy.
- Exercise. When you exercise at a mild or moderate intensity, you'll feel calmer and less hungry. You'll heighten your endorphins too. So choose a fun exercise and try it even if you don't feel like it. The payoff is worth it.

▪ THE ANTI-PMS CUSTOMIZER ▪

The cure for PMS begins at the breakfast table. Studies confirm that what, when, and how you eat has a direct effect on the nature and severity of your symptoms. Follow the Power-Up Food Plan (chapter 7) and emphasize the following:

1. Eat anti-PMS foods.

When PMS symptoms hit, particularly moodiness or irritability, choose anti-PMS foods and avoid foods that aggravate PMS. Here are examples.

ANTI-PMS FOODS	PMS-AGGRAVATING FOODS
High-fiber carbos, including bread, bagels, and grains; vegetables and fruits	Meat
B_6-rich foods, such as whole grains, nuts, and legumes	Cheese
Sweet-creamy treats in moderation, especially chocolate	Fat-heavy snacks in large portions, such as several slices of deep-dish pizza or three scoops of ultrarich ice cream

2. Eat anti-PMS foods at the right times.

The right time is any time you feel moody, blue, tense, or "off." An exception: If you have PMS symptoms and feel calm, eating carbos alone may make you drowsy. To sidestep drowsiness, eat a carbo-protein mix.

3. Eat anti-PMS foods in the right combos.

Eat carbos alone (usually—see exception above) and B_6-rich foods anytime.

Anti-PMS tip of the day: When you feel moody, stop by an ice cream parlor, order a single-scoop of your favorite flavor, and enjoy without guilt.

■ THE FOOD BLUES ■

When Bill has a beer, his thoughts darken. "When I drink alcohol, I want to retreat and crawl into a shell," says the Chicagoan. Curiously, Bill and thousands of other food-mood sufferers experience depression because of what they eat. It could be the milk poured on their breakfast cereal or the eggs in last night's omelette or any number of foods.

Sometimes a food-mood sufferer may feel emotions like anger, nervousness, or even giddiness. Most typically, a food-mood sufferer feels "blue" or "burned out," though everything else in life seems fine: His spouse is attentive, the kids are healthy, and work is going smoothly.

The culprits—and the cure—often lie within arm's reach. In cupboards. In pantries. In refrigerators.

It seems ironic that food, meant to sustain us and nourish us, can contribute to depression, or "the blues," like in Bill's case. But it makes sense: Research shows that foods can help us change a blue mood, medicating us with serotonin and the endorphins, making us feel "normal" again. So if foods can enhance our moods, surely they can worsen them too.

The million-dollar question is, How can you determine whether food is making you blue and, if so, what should you do?

Take this quickie quiz to help you find out:

Do you feel irritable, anxious, or depressed after eating any of the following foods? (Check all that apply.)

Alcohol _____	*Meat (red meat or poultry)* _____
Candy _____	*Milk* _____
Chocolate _____	*Oats* _____
Citrus _____	*Soft drinks (regular)* _____
Coffee _____	*Soft drinks (containing aspartame)* _____
Corn _____	*Soy* _____
Eggs _____	*Sugar* _____
Fish _____	*Wheat* _____
Grapes _____	

Look over the above list of probable suspect foods, which research has shown to cause food-mood disorders in some people, and eliminate all the ones you checked from your diet for a week. At the end of the week, ask yourself: "Do I feel happier, less tense, more hopeful, better in general?" If so, chances are one or more of the foods you checked blues your mood.

If eliminating your suspect foods makes no difference in your mood, you may still be eating a food that's eating away at happiness. You just haven't yet identified it. Look over the list again, adjust your meals if appropriate, and note your mood, or follow a strict elimination diet.

Once you've eliminated your suspect foods *and* observed marked improvement in your mood, add one of them back to your diet. Now how do you feel? Worse? Eliminate the food again for three days and see whether your good mood returns. If so, keep the suspect food out of your diet. If adding back the food made no difference in your mood, you probably can continue eating it with no ill effects.

Repeat this same food test with every suspect food you checked.

Before we go on, let me offer this insight. Some people are unaware of a food's effect on their mood. They just happen to be less sensitive to mood changes than other people. But a suspect food may still be at the heart of their bad mood.

If this sounds like you— or if you just want to be certain one way or the

A TRUE FOOD ALLERGY?

It's well known that allergies to food or any irritant like pollen or ragweed can cause physical reactions like hives, digestive problems, sneezing, and difficult breathing. Now some researchers are blaming food allergies for fatigue, mood swings, and anxiety too.

Their studies remain controversial.

Some people confuse food allergies with adverse food reactions. For instance, lactose intolerance may cause bloating, abdominal pain, and diarrhea, but the symptoms are caused by a lack of the enzyme lactase, which breaks down milk sugar for digestion.

A true food allergy involves the immune system. Its job is to protect the body from invaders, and it may sometimes think a morsel of food is a danger. Body substances including immunoglobulin E (IgE), basophils, and mast cells join in the attack. The result: an allergic response.

Among the most common allergy-inducing foods are peanuts, walnuts, wheat, soy, corn, tomatoes, strawberries, oranges, eggs, and milk. Children who develop food allergies often grow out of them. Usually, an adult's reaction to food is caused by an intolerance, not an allergy.

In either case, here's what you can do if you suspect a food allergy or intolerance.

Go on a modified diet. Based on your current knowledge of past experiences, make a list of the foods that seem to cause you uncomfortable physical or psychological symptoms. Then stop eating all of these foods for at least a week. If you don't feel better, you may still be eating a food causing you problems. In this case, try the elimination diet, detailed below.

If you do feel better on the modified diet, add back a suspect food for a few days and note how you feel. Fine? Then keep it in your diet. Worse? Avoid it altogether and test another suspect food. Most important, test one food at a time and let a few days pass between tests.

Follow the elimination diet when you are unsure which foods trigger symptoms of allergy or intolerance. First, remove the most common allergen-causing foods listed on the previous page, along with chocolate, fish, and shellfish. Because some people have mold allergies, you should also eliminate foods prone to mold growth, including cheese, mushrooms, yogurt, wine, and beer.

Keep them out of your diet for a week and note how you feel. If you do not feel better, seek the expertise of a doctor or other health practitioner. He or she can recommend more specific food tests and monitor your progress.

More than likely, on the elimination diet, you will see the disappearance of many if not all of your symptoms. Now add back a suspect food for a few days. If you feel fine, keep it in your diet. If you feel worse, figure that you have an allergy or intolerance to the food and stop eating it. Continue these tests of a single food at a time, waiting a couple of days in between tests, until you've checked out all suspect foods.

Do not stay on an elimination diet indefinitely, because it may lack variety and create nutritional deficiencies.

other—follow the strict elimination diet detailed in "A True Food Allergy?" on page 77.

Thousands of case histories of food-mood sufferers are recorded, yet some scientists still wonder whether their disorder is psychologically or biologically based. If the cause is psychological, with some food-mood sufferers erroneously blaming their diet for emotional difficulties, then they do indeed need help. And, quite likely, a percentage of food-mood sufferers do fall in this camp.

But there's growing evidence for a biological link. Apparently, food-mood sufferers may have food intolerances, reactions, or allergies that trigger the blues. While there is some controversy over this subject—for instance, a person who says she has a reaction to a particular food does not show symptoms in a controlled test—some evidence suggests that food sensitivities are to blame.

For instance, in a study at the University of Chicago, researchers administered capsules of wheat, milk, chocolate, and a placebo (a placebo is a look-alike capsule designed to have no effect) to twenty-three psychiatric patients who claimed to have emotional reactions to food. They also gave the capsules to twelve nonpatients who claimed not to have reactions. The participants underwent evaluations of behavior, psychiatric factors, and blood tests.

The results showed that sixteen of the psychiatric patients (and none of the other subjects) experienced marked mood changes—depression, anxiety, and irritability—from wheat and milk but not chocolate.

Though this study was small and more research is needed for confirmation, a biological basis for the blues brought on by food seems legitimate. Biochemists already know that food affects your neurotransmitters, which determine your mood—for better, for worse.

A BLACK HOLE

Anyone can suffer the darkness of depression. The term *depression* is commonly used to refer to mild moodiness, utter anguish, and every downer emotion in between. But clinical depression is a disease that interferes with normal functioning.

Some warning signs:

- a change in sleeping habits (insomnia or waking before dawn)
- a change in eating habits (such as a loss in appetite)
- a loss of usual interests
- an inability to concentrate
- feelings of worthlessness or guilt
- a lack of energy
- overwhelming feelings of sadness and anxiety
- suicidal thoughts or attempted suicide

Estimates claim that some fifty million Americans will suffer from depression—whether mild, moderate, or severe—at some point in their lives. Contrary to common belief, people who suffer depression cannot "snap out of it." Their condition is real and often more disabling than many other ailments taken more seriously, such as high blood pressure and diabetes.

I'll be the last to claim that what you eat can cure clinical depression. If you have any, and certainly more than three, of the warning signs, you ought to get professional help right away. Depression can be treated successfully with psychotherapy, medication, or a combination.

Though power-eating is no replacement for medical care, it can help. So hang in there and listen up, especially if you're not clinically depressed but suffer "the blues," which can be defined as feeling kind of sad or melancholy or just not quite right.

To see how food chases away the blues, let's revisit the "comforting" neurotransmitter, serotonin.

DO YOU NEED EXPERT HELP?

When facing a very difficult time (a divorce, a serious illness, the grief of losing a loved one, the remembrance of a painful childhood), your mood may hit the skids. You may feel any number of depression symptoms: irritability, anger, sadness, fatigue, lethargy, insomnia, overeating or undereating, emotional numbness, hopelessness, and/or helplessness.

Following the Power-Up Food Plan won't make your emotional or physical pain vanish, but it can help keep you in a better mood than if you ate poorly.

However, if your depression symptoms have lasted more than two weeks or are moderate to severe, or if you have had suicidal thoughts or urges, consult your doctor or health practitioner immediately. A medical examination may uncover a physical cause for your depression. If a physical cause is ruled out, he or she may point you toward therapy, medication, a support group, or a combination.

Remember, depression is not a sign of weakness. It's a signal that you need to reach out and get help. The sooner, the better.

ANOTHER SEROTONIN SERENADE

By now you know serotonin is a mood regulator extraordinaire. When you've got the right amount, your mood will be optimal. Of course, optimal functioning doesn't mean you'll never get down or cry. I mean, if you lose your job or your granddad dies, you ought to feel sad or angry or frustrated. That's normal. Feeling emotions means you've got mood power.

The difference between having the right amount of serotonin and too little is profound. When you have the right amount and you lose your job, for instance, you bounce back more quickly. You have the desire and energy to get your résumé together and start looking for new employment. You have hope. You may even discover legitimate reasons for why a new job may be in your best interest.

Having low serotonin is a troublesome tale. Losing your job shrouds your world in darkness. You ruminate over why you got fired and how it shows you're a loser. You fear job hunting because you might get rejected, confirming the erroneous belief that you'll "fail" again. Your energy wanes. You know there's something wrong inside. But what?

What's wrong may be your low serotonin level—and quite possibly your inadequate intake of blues-busting nutrients.

As mentioned, the best drug-free way to boost serotonin levels is by eating complex carbos without protein whenever you feel tense, jittery, fatigued, sad, blah, or just not right. When you follow my Power-Up Food Plan (chapter 7), this phenomenon will occur naturally. But you can almost guarantee a good mood by increasing your intake of several key nutrients. Very often psychological symptoms of a marginal deficiency show up before physical warning signs.

We've looked at them in previous chapters. Here's a quick refresher.

Vitamin B$_6$: Depressed people are likely to have a B$_6$ deficiency, research shows. This vitamin is integral to the manufacture of serotonin. Recommended dietary allowance (RDA): 1.6 milligrams (mg) for women; 2mg for men.

Folic acid: Another B vitamin, folic acid helps ward off the blues. In a study of healthy people, those with the highest levels had the best moods, while those with "low-normal" blood levels were more likely to be depressed. RDA: 180 micrograms (mcg) for women; 200mcg for men.

Vitamin B$_{12}$: Marginal intake of this vitamin is also linked to depression. It's found only in animal foods like dairy products and eggs, fortified foods, and nutritional supplements. RDA: 2mcg for men and women.

Minerals: Research shows that a diet low in any one of several minerals—iron, magnesium, zinc, and calcium—may bring on the blues. Be sure to get the Recommended Dietary Allowance; supplement as necessary.

The bottom line: Stay away from foods that make you blue, load up on nutrient-rich cuisine, and eat complex carbos usually and a sweet-creamy treat occasionally, if desired, when you're feeling emotions ranging from anguish to blah. And, without a doubt, get professional help when you or a loved one thinks there may be a chance that you need it.

▪ THE BLUES-BUSTER CUSTOMIZER ▪

You can feel better by power-eating and staying away from foods that trigger a bad mood. Of course, the blues, the melancholy that grays your day, differs from clinical depression. Clinical depression requires medical care, though power-eating may improve some symptoms of clinical depression.

1. *Eat blues-buster foods and avoid super-blue foods.* Here are examples.

BLUES-BUSTER FOODS	SUPER-BLUE FOODS
Any carbo eaten alone, except for those that trigger a bad mood.	Foods that trigger a bad mood. Likely culprits include wheat, corn, soy, milk, eggs, peanuts, and citrus.
Foods rich in B vitamins, including legumes, whole grains, nuts, vegetables, fruits, dairy products and eggs, but avoid those that trigger a bad mood.	High-fat meals Junk food

2. *Eat blues-buster foods at the right time.*
Power-eating all the time is a good defense against the blues. When they hit, go for a carbo-only meal or snack except when you feel tired.

3. *Eat blues-buster foods in the right combos.*

Carbos only, except when you're tired. When you need an energy boost, eat protein alone or a protein-carbo mix.

Blues-buster tip of the day: If your blue mood persists or intensifies, seek medical help pronto.

BY THE WAY

My research turned up a curious tidbit: Eating meat apparently does not contribute to the blues. I could locate no studies indicating a meat-depression link.

However, common sense dictates that choosing nutritional foods regularly may improve your health and your outlook on life. Just the other day I received reassuring E-mail from a new vegetarian who says she had suffered depression for years. In the past year since opting for vegetarian cuisine day in and day out, she reports making more progress than in the ten previous years combined.

"All I know is I feel better," she says. "I have been much calmer, more rational, and more in control of my emotions. Everyone close to me has noticed the difference in my attitude and personality—my therapist, my parents, my friends.

"I am completely sold that the vegetarian diet is the best one."

POWER QUIZ

In Need of a Better Mood?

Everyone has blue days on occasion. That's perfectly normal. So is feeling nervous before giving a speech, taking an exam, or competing in a sport. In contrast, being stuck in a continual funk, experiencing wild mood swings, or feeling intense anger, guilt, shame, or other downer emotions is not healthy.

To get a sense of your need for a mood boost, answer yes or no to these questions.

1. Do you have more happy days than blue days?
   _____ yes   _____ no

2. When you feel blue, or depressed, do you turn to food for comfort?   _____ yes   _____ no

3. Do you think anger is a bad emotion?
   _____ yes   _____ no

4. Do you occasionally go into rages or give others "the quiet treatment" when you're angry?
   _____ yes   _____ no

5. Do you eat at least eight servings of grains each day?
   _____ yes   _____ no

6. When you get a craving or a desire for a carbo like bread, mashed potatoes, chocolate, or ice cream, do you usually eat your desired goodie?   _____ yes   _____ no

7. When you eat your desired goodie, do you eat a lot of it?
   _____ yes   _____ no

8. Do you regularly engage in aerobic exercise?
   _____ yes   _____ no

9. Do you often feel stressed out?
   _____ yes   _____ no

10. Do you have high blood pressure?
    _____ yes   _____ no

11. Do you talk to a supportive mate or friend when you have a problem?   _____ yes   _____ no

12. Would you describe yourself as usually energetic?
    _____ yes   _____ no

13. Would you describe yourself as usually tense?
    _____ yes   _____ no

14. Do you often enjoy moments of play, such as roughhousing with the kids, going sledding or snowmobiling, or jumping in a pile of leaves?   _____ yes   _____ no

15. Do you have enough time for yourself?

_____ yes _____ no

16. Do you often feel fatigued?

_____ yes _____ no

17. Do you have trouble falling asleep?

_____ yes _____ no

18. Do you take a moderate-dose vitamin and mineral supplement daily or almost daily?

_____ yes _____ no

19. Do you avoid fat-heavy meals?

_____ yes _____ no

20. Are you in general good-to-excellent health?

_____ yes _____ no

Give yourself one point for each yes answer to questions 1, 5, 6, 8, 11, 12, 14, 15, 18, 19, and 20, and for each no answer to questions 2, 3, 4, 7, 9, 10, 13, 16, and 17. The highest possible score is 20.

If you scored 17 to 20 points, you're making excellent good-mood choices and, subsequently, are probably feeling just fine almost always.

A score of 12 to 16 points suggests that you have times of stress and/or tenseness that can interfere with achieving an optimal mood. You also experience times of good mood.

Fewer than 12 points? Begin power-eating for a better mood and making other positive lifestyle choices to feel your best.

In any case, if you become depressed, anxious, or have another psychological problem that persists or is intense, seek medical help promptly. You can be helped.

Do You Have a
Food Craving?

You're stuck in traffic when all of a sudden a food craving strikes. It comes quick. It comes strong. It comes like a panther on the prowl. And the prey? It's you.

The craving may be for a Snickers bar, a danish, chocolate, Chunky Monkey, or french fries. Or perhaps you ache for strawberries, carrot juice, freshly baked multi-grain bread, or another nutritional saint.

Up the road sits a 7-Eleven, beckoning.

What should you do?

A. Try your very, very best to ignore your food craving.

B. Proceed to the 7-Eleven and fulfill it.

If you selected *B,* you made the wise choice. Fulfilling your biological food cravings, which differ from emotional food cravings, as you'll hear in a few moments, is smart because you're listening to your body. When you heed the vital messages sent by your brain to eat a certain type of food, you are power-eating and will feel, think, and perform better.

For instance, research suggests that carbo-cravers tend to have lower serotonin levels than people who prefer protein-rich snacks. Their lower serotonin levels may prompt them to raid the cookie jar as a way to counter anxiety, depression, and irritability. By eating a few cookies, carbo-cravers in need of a serotonin "fix" can boost their mood and feel better overall.

By definition, a biological food craving is a nutritional need for a certain type of food to balance brain chemicals. Remember the neurotransmitters serotonin, dopamine, norepinephrine, the endorphins, and neuropeptide Y? These and other body chemicals trigger biological food cravings.

New research is showing that when you fulfill your biological food cravings, you can experience the following:

- high spirits
- calm nerves
- energy
- better concentration
- clearer and quicker thinking
- improved memory
- heightened physical performance

And what happens if you pooh-pooh your biological food cravings? Not only will you miss out on the power-eating benefits mentioned above, but you may also set yourself up for a poor mood, a muddled mind, and a body breakdown, with colds and flus a likely bed partner. Plus, when you deny your biological food cravings, you'll be an easy victim for an all-out, no-holds-barred food binge.

It's deliciously true: Your favorite forbidden foods may actually be good for you. So forget willpower. It rarely works.

Sure, you might "just say no" to your beloved Dove bars for a week, maybe even a month or two. But sooner or later, your willpower will collapse like a chocolate soufflé. Chances are, you'll fall hard, gobbling up Dove bars in record speed.

Just don't feel guilty.

When your body needs carbos to counteract a bad mood, or protein to stop fuzzy thinking, or fat to ease the pain of PMS, it will demand obedience. You have no choice but to give in to your biological food cravings.

The goal is to work with, not against, these cravings and feel good again.

▪ THE TWO TYPES OF CRAVINGS ▪

The dictionary defines *craving* this way: an intense, urgent, or abnormal desire or longing.

Intense, yes. Urgent, yes. Abnormal? No way.

As mentioned, a biological food craving is a *normal* need for a specific food that can give you power—mood, brain, and body power. The trick is figuring out whether your food craving is biological or emotional—or both.

Here are two clues.

When you have a biological food craving and fulfill it, you feel nourished. It doesn't take much food to meet your biological needs either. One bagel, a wedge or two of low-fat cheese, or a couple of chocolates—that's it.

In contrast, emotional eating is looking for comfort in food. It's often brought on by "I'm a loser" thinking. And a small treat is never enough. Never.

I think of a sad story a friend I'll call Paula told me.

Years ago, Paula was a stay-at-home mom with young children, struggling with boredom, stress, and a negative self-image. To please her family, she'd occasionally bake a chocolate cake, with every intention of saving it for the evening's dessert.

One morning before Paula's husband left for work, she told him to expect his favorite homemade cake when he returned. While her little ones napped, she baked and frosted it and licked the bowls clean. She set her creation on the kitchen counter and curled up on the sofa to relax.

Within a minute, she sensed the proverbial devil and angel, one on her left shoulder, the other on her right. She says their conversation went something like this:

"Go ahead and cut yourself a slice," whispered the devil to

Paula. "A few forkfuls won't wreck your diet, and you deserve a treat."

"Don't listen to him," said the angel. "He's the father of lies. If you eat one slice, you might eat another, then another, just like last time. Care for yourself by listening to your true need: love. Food can't replace it."

But the devil wouldn't let up. "C'mon, one little slice is— what? three hundred and fifty measly calories?" he said. "You know you want it. You can stop eating any time you choose. You'll feel better, I promise, Paula."

The devil won this battle. With pictures of chocolate cake dancing in her eyes, Paula walked into the kitchen as if in a trance. She ate a slice, cut another and shoveled it in, then a third. When half of the cake was gone, guilt overwhelmed her. She could barely believe she'd eaten so much, so fast.

Inside Paula wept tears of shame. She hurled insults at herself. "You slob," she told herself. "You have no self-control. You're disgusting. You deserve to feel rotten." And she did, physically and emotionally.

To her mind, she had one solution: Bake another chocolate cake, just like the first, to hide her "crime." But she had to do it fast. Her kids would wake soon. Now what to do with the extra half cake? Eat it, Paula concluded. That would be the cleanest way to dispose of the incriminating evidence of her binge. She did, hating herself all the more with each forkful.

Paula's story is tragic and too common. Medical centers with diet programs like the one at Duke University in Durham, North Carolina, scores of weight-loss books, and Overeaters Anonymous help emotional eaters uncover the real reasons why they overeat.

■ SPOONING FOR LOVE ■

Emotional eaters confuse love and self-acceptance with food and often comfort themselves with their coveted goodies. Food is their drug of choice.

Lonely? Spooning in a huge bowl of ice cream seems a safe "friend." Anxious? Crunching a king-size bag of chips can give nervous hands something to do. Angry? Eating any food in excess can be a distraction and a way to "stuff" feelings—until self-hate slithers to the fore.

But food is a poor substitute for love of self, others, and God (or whatever name an emotional eater attaches to her Higher Power).

Some emotional eaters barely eat at all. Remember Karen Carpenter? An anorexic, she starved herself into the grave, believing that thinness equaled happiness. Sadly, the scene repeats among many girls and women throughout the Western world. (More on eating disorders, including anorexia nervosa and bulimia nervosa, in "When Food Becomes an Enemy".)

To be fair, some people who overeat may not be emotional eaters. For instance, businesspeople who regularly entertain clients may pack on pounds if they frequent restaurants ped-

---

WHEN FOOD BECOMES AN ENEMY

Linda is skin and bones and diets to lose more weight, mistakenly believing she's fat. Dee seems a healthy weight but routinely binges on sweets and self-induces vomiting. Gale stuffs herself with food, though what she really wants is love.

These three women, whose names have been changed, suffer from eating disorders. In the past decade, the number of people with disorders has increased about 50 percent. Some have anorexia nervosa, in which they eat so little that they face near starvation. Others have bulimia nervosa, in which they binge and purge by vomiting or using laxatives. Still others are chronic overeaters.

Though a healthy vegetarian diet is an excellent way to maintain a proper weight and avoid killer diseases like heart disease and some cancers, some people tag themselves as vegetarian to rationalize rigid food choices. A college student, for instance, may pass up not only meat but also the variety of vegetarian foods she needs for health, saying something like, "I couldn't eat [fill-in-the-blank]. It has far too much fat."

Power-eating combined with medical intervention, including psychological counseling as necessary, can restore good eating habits. Power-eating helps to balance body chemicals, which may no longer act properly after erratic eating habits like starvation and bingeing.

A hormonelike subtance called cholecystokinin (CCK), for instance, which controls the body's hunger-satiety system, may not kick in for bulimics but tell anorexics that they're full after a nibble or two of food. Fortunately, eating right again and gaining weight can normalize the workings of CCK. In addition, serotonin levels may be low in bulimics and the endorphins out of whack in both bulimics and anorexics. Again, power-eating is one key to normalizing brain chemicals.

Some warning signs of eating disorders:

Loss of 15 percent of normal body
weight

Frequent weighing

Preoccupation with calorie counting

Disturbed sleep

Secretive behavior

Frequent vomiting or use of laxatives

Fatigue

Difficulty concentrating

Distorted self-image

dling rich fare and large portions. Ex-athletes may get fat too. They're in the habit of forking in the huge meals of their heyday in sports, but now aren't exercising regularly to burn off the excess calories.

As mentioned, emotional eating differs from biological food cravings in one extremely important way: Emotional eating is eating in response to a mood; fulfilling a biological food craving is eating in response to your neurotransmitters. Mood versus neurotransmitters—that's the difference.

But as you might imagine, emotional eaters may suffer depression, anxiety, or other ills and may turn to food not only for comfort but also to balance brain chemicals. So in one sense they are eating to supply their bodies with what it biologically craves.

The problem is, emotional eaters may stay at the table long after they've given themselves enough food to meet their biological needs. The body only needs a small amount of certain foods—say, one or two ounces—to affect the neurotransmitters.

If you eat compulsively or as a way to deal with emotions, I hope you see the red warning flags and get help. Consider psychological counseling, including cognitive therapy, stress reduction, exercise, and twelve-step groups.

And power-eat too. Power-eating helps to stabilize your moods and increases the chances you'll put emotional eating in your past and learn to respect your biological food cravings.

First, embrace the truth that satisfying your biological cravings—whether for carbos, protein, or fat—makes you a power-eater.

Second, choose a moderate portion of exactly what you crave and feel no guilt.

Not a twinge.

▪ HUNGRY FOR NEUROTRANSMITTERS ▪

When Steve wakes up, his body shouts, "Carbos, carbos, and more carbos," and in response to his biological food craving, he pours himself a big bowl of Cheerios.

More than likely, you eat carbos in the morning too, thanks to neurotransmitter neuropeptide Y, or NPY for short. As your blood glucose level drops during sleep, NPY courses through your body and demands carbos. This is why toast, waffles, pancakes, and cornflakes are breakfast favorites.

Your body—or, more specifically, NPY—passes messages to your brain cells that you need a carbo boost. When you eat carbos, preferably complex carbos like whole grains, your digestive enzymes break them down into glucose molecules, which speed to your brain. Your brain needs a constant supply of glucose for optimal functioning.

What would happen if Steve were to choose a plateful of scrambled eggs over carbos? This low-carbo breakfast would not fulfill his biological food craving. Chances are, he would succumb to a midmorning treat of frosted doughnuts.

The good news: The sweet treats are carbo-rich. Finally, Steve's brain would be getting the glucose it needs.

The bad news: Sugar weighs down these sweet treats. It would seat him on a roller coaster of high and low blood sugar levels and create more sugar cravings that can mess with his mind, emotions, and body. (See "The Sugar Boogie Blues," page 41.)

▪ CARBO CRAVINGS ▪

My author-friend Victoria noticed a curious connection between her occasional bouts of anxiety-producing writer's block and carrot juice. When she couldn't write, she ached for a glass of this naturally sweet elixir.

Carrot juice is almost pure carbos. Eight ounces boasts 23 grams of carbohydrates and a load of beta-carotene, known to be a potent antioxidant. It's exactly what her body needs to calm

her down, to help her focus, and to increase her ability to concentrate whenever writer's block strikes.

Says Victoria, "It's like a blood transfusion. It picks me up in
an instant."

Notice that her body knew what it needed: the carbos in the
carrot juice. As described in the previous chapters, eating carbos
in absence of protein causes increases in blood levels of glucose
and the hormone insulin. Insulin ushers several amino acids except tryptophan into the body's cells, letting tryptophan speed to
the brain where it helps manufacture serotonin, the "comforting"
neurotransmitter.

Picture it this way:

*anxiety → desire for carbos → eat carbos → increase of
brain level of tryptophan → increase of serotonin →
greater calm and productivity*

Biological cravings for carbos can hit not only when you're
anxious but also when you're depressed or blue. (See the previous
chapter.) Carbo cravings also pop up in the morning, during emotional or physical stress, and/or during restrictive dieting.

When fulfilling a biological craving for carbos, choose complex carbos (whole grains, vegetables, fruits) over simple carbos
(candy, cake, Popsicles)—usually.

As long as you don't have a medical reason to avoid them
entirely (diabetes, for instance), a small amount of sweet nothings
probably won't trigger the sugar boogie blues. Even better, to
slow the rise in blood sugar, eat your small snack with complex
carbos or a bit of fat.

A few snack suggestions: jam (simple carbo) on whole-wheat
toast (complex carbo); a cookie (simple carbo and fat); sherbet
(simple carbo) following a vegetable sauté with brown rice (complex carbo); and half a chocolate bar (simple carbo and fat). You
get the idea.

But suppose you usually crave protein. If this sounds like you,
I have a question: Do you wear boxers?

■ PROTEIN OR BUST ■

In *Why Women Need Chocolate,* author Debra Waterhouse shares some interesting results about American men and women and their food cravings. She compiled the results from six hundred respondents. Here's what she found.

COMPARED TO WOMEN, MEN ARE...	COMPARED TO MEN, WOMEN ARE...
78% more likely to crave meat	76% more likely to crave chocolate
76% more likely to crave eggs	71% more likely to crave crackers
69% more likely to crave hot dogs	62% more likely to crave ice cream
10% more likely to crave pizza	62% more likely to crave candy
10% more likely to crave seafood	65% more likely to crave fruit

These are striking differences. The men in general desired protein to the max, while the women said, "Thanks, but no thanks. We'll take the carbos and fat."

As Waterhouse and other nutrition researchers reason, men biologically need and crave more protein than do women because they have more testosterone and greater muscle mass. In contrast, women biologically need and crave more carbos and fat than do men because they have more estrogen and body fat.

Not surprisingly, far more women than men dine exclusively on vegetarian cuisine. Though vegetarians eat ample protein, easily meeting the Recommended Dietary Allowance for this nutrient, their protein sources are primarily vegetable-based. Most American vegetarians and almost vegetarians also include eggs and dairy foods at some meals.

Though protein-cravers usually are men, the intense, urgent longing for a meat-free Boca Burger, with 14 grams of protein per two-and-one-half-ounce patty, can strike anyone, anytime.

For instance, Karen Cope Straus, a former managing editor of *Vegetarian Times,* admitted in print that she became a protein packer.

It all started with a story assignment to devise a vegetarian "zone" eating plan, which a number of the magazine's readers had requested. *The Zone,* a book by Barry Sears, Ph.D., promoting what became a phenomenally popular and controversial fad diet of the midnineties, recommends a diet heavy on protein and light on carbos.

Sears claims most Americans overload their plates with pasta, bread, potatoes, rice, and sweets, creating imbalances in insulin levels that may result in disease. In other words, he believes that the real culprit behind your health problems, including the spare tire around your middle if you have one, is a high-carbo diet.

Scientists on the whole and health organizations

---

7 WAYS TO HANDLE CRAVINGS

The best way to handle a biological craving is to fulfill it. Promptly. Biological cravings clue you in on what your body needs—a certain nutrient, a boost in blood sugar, a balance in brain chemicals.

To get control of your cravings, so you keep on power-eating, try these suggestions:

1. Eat a breakfast rich in complex carbos. Your body is programmed to desire carbos after a night of sleep.
2. Be a grazer. Instead of eating three big meals, have five or six smaller ones spaced throughout the day.
3. Reduce your sugar intake. When you shovel in sugar, your mood perks up then plummets. Choose complex carbos like a bagel or low-fat muffin.
4. Avoid artificial sweeteners. Trying to trick your taste buds into believing you're eating sugar when you're not can backfire, setting you up for a binge.
5. Be present. While eating a food you crave, don't read a book, watch TV, or drive the car. Fully enjoy the food and feel satisfied.
6. Don't eat to squelch emotions. When you do so, you become an emotional eater; you're not fulfilling a biological food craving. Learn to deal with your emotions directly.
7. Splurge sometimes. If you want three scoops of ice cream, though you know one would suffice, treat yourself. The worst thing you can do is to become rigid.

---

like the American Dietetic Association have panned Sears's claims. Yet the get-thin-quick public ate it up, as did *Vegetarian Times*'s former managing editor Straus.

She followed her own vegetarian-adapted zone diet, with Sears's recommended ratio of 40 percent of calories from carbos, 30 percent from protein, and 30 percent from fat. By the way, federal nutrition guidelines call for 10 to 15 percent of calories from protein.

Straus says her zone-adapted diet helped her lose weight and gain energy. Even her nails and hair seemed healthier to her.

Before you "zone out," keep this in mind: Sears's fad diet restricts calories, which triggers weight loss, but has so much protein that it may bring on ketosis, a metabolic disturbance. His diet also pushes nutrient-rich veggies like broccoli and spinach in lieu of complex carbos like whole-wheat bread. It plainly lacks variety, a key to power-eating and good health in general.

But please do savor a protein-rich snack whenever you have a biological craving for protein. It may signal a need for increased dopamine and norepinephrine, both "alertness" neurotransmitters manufactured from the amino acid tyrosine. Tyrosine teems in protein-rich foods, including low-fat dairy products, eggs, legumes, and soy foods like textured vegetable protein.

eat protein-rich foods (alone or with carbos) to avoid carbo overload → *increase of brain level of tyrosine* → *increase of dopamine and norepinephrine* → *mental, emotional, and physical acuity*

Here's the interesting question: Since vegetarians and almost vegetarians eat ample protein, why would we—or anyone—get a biological craving for protein? One reason makes sense: We may crave protein due to carbo overload.

If you eat lots of carbos without protein-rich foods when you're already calm and content, your serotonin levels rise sharply. Sounds great, but it ain't. Too much serotonin makes you drowsy, mentally lethargic, fuzzy-headed, and "off."

Protein cravings can stop carbo overload.

My friend John, an almost vegetarian with an easygoing manner, eats protein at every meal and says he feels great almost all the time. He doesn't crunch numbers to figure out his daily intake of protein grams. It's just the way he eats because it feels right. He listens to his body and gives it what it needs—even when it says it wants some fats.

■ GO FOR GALANIN ■

Who hasn't craved potato chips or ice cream or chocolate or buttered bread on occasion?

Lora, a woman with hair the color of dark chocolate and a contagious smile, certainly does. Her favorite is chocolate. She doesn't need scientific proof that this sweet provides an impeccable pick-me-up.

"I usually have a piece or two of chocolate early in the afternoon after a busy, stressful morning," says Lora, a mother of four kids under age nine. "I feel pampered after my sweet treat. I feel good. And just a little is all I need."

Spoken like a true biological food craver!

Your body has a built-in appetite for endorphin-happy fat too. Specifically, the neurotransmitter galanin is like a maitre d' who directs you to a table and seduces you with the specials of the day. Along with neuropeptide Y, galanin is a main appetite regulator. As the day progresses, your galanin levels rise, urging you to eat higher-fat foods. Typically galanin levels peak in the late afternoon through the evening.

Galanin goes hand in hand with the endorphins. In fact, they coexist in the same nerve cells. Researchers believe that galanin may turn on biological food cravings for fat while the endorphins add delicious pleasure to its fulfilling.

Some studies show that trying to restrict your intake of fat may cause rebound. That's right: You may end up bingeing on a box of chocolate chip cookies, a pint of Häagen-Dazs, and a half-dozen Twinkies when you don't listen to your biological cravings for fat.

Am I condoning eating as much fat as you want anytime you want? Yes and no.

As I've been saying in this chapter, listen to your biological food cravings. If your neurotransmitters say, "Hey, have a scoop of Chunky Monkey," eat that small amount and enjoy it without hesitation or guilt. Remember, you have the power to say no once you've had your fill, and there's no physiological reason to go overboard.

■ HANDLING SPECIAL CRAVINGS ■

Pregnant? Menopausal? Got PMS or S.A.D.?

If so, you've had special cravings. During these times, your brain calls out for certain foods, sometimes carbos, sometimes protein, sometimes fat.

Baby and me. Stories of husbands driving late at night to buy ice cream and pickles for their pregnant wives are legendary. If you or your mate have ever been pregnant, you probably have some hilarious memories.

I remember my mom's stories about her cravings for hot fudge sundaes that would pop up out of nowhere only minutes before the nearby ice cream parlor closed for the night. She begged my dad to get her a goodie and drove him nuts for the better part of nine months.

While nutrition researchers believe that food cravings during pregnancy signal the body's physiological need for calories and nutrients, another factor may be at work: a pregnant woman's desire to involve her spouse and friends in her pregnancy.

Scientists agree, however, that pregnancy and food cravings go together like bread and butter, especially during the first trimester, with fluctuations in many body chemicals, including hormones and neurotransmitters.

The change—for the better. During menopause, marked by the cessation of a woman's menstrual cycle, food cravings and aversions are the norm. A woman who once ate whole-grain breads may now want boxed macaroni and cheese. Another can't get enough milk, a food she rarely drank before menopause. As in pregnancy, the reasons for food cravings have everything to do with hormonal changes and neurotransmitters.

Your cravings before and after menopause may differ significantly too. After menopause, for instance, you may notice that you no longer crave fat and sugar. Instead, you want vegetables, fruit, and protein. How come?

After menopause, estrogen and other hormones no longer rise and fall each month, and so do not affect brain chemicals as dramatically. Also, with estrogen now a minor player, testosterone (the "male" hormone, which all women possess a bit of) has a stronger influence on the female body, possibly explaining the protein cravings.

The moody blues. PMS and S.A.D., which stand for premenstrual syndrome and seasonal affective disorder, respectively, bring on food cravings—and how!

> ### THE NEW BABY BLUES
>
> In the first week or so after your baby made his grand debut, did you feel weepy, discontented, or anxious? About half of all new mothers do. The baby blues seem to be caused by the drop in endorphins after childbirth.
>
> Usually the baby blues clear up within a few days, though sometimes it may last for six weeks or, in a smaller percentage, for months. The long-lasting baby blues is true postpartum depression.
>
> It passes with time, but who wants to wait? You see other new moms cuddling their newborns with an obvious look of joy on their faces while you may want to hide under your bed covers. In addition to getting rest, asking for help with chores and with the baby, making time for yourself, getting out of the house, and seeking professional help, if needed, you should power-eat.
>
> When you eat foods to affect your brain chemistry—in short, protein for alertness, carbos for calm, and a little fat for feel-good sensations—you can make a bad mood better. See the Power-Up Food Plan (Chapter 7).
>
> If at any time you get an urge to harm your baby, go to a neighbor's home and call someone who can get to you right away—your husband, a family member, or a friend—and phone your doctor or 911. You can be helped.

As you heard in the previous chapter, PMS is tied up with fluctuations in your hormones and neurotransmitters. In the week or two before menstruation, a woman typically ups her calorie intake, much of it from carbos. Likewise, people saddled with S.A.D., a type of depression that appears in the gray winter months, also crave carbos because of a need for increased serotonin.

So what should you do if you're pregnant, menopausal, PMSing, or have S.A.D., and a biological food craving hits you strong and fast like a panther on the prowl?

I think you know the answer by now.

Fulfill it and recharge your mood, mind, and body. And repeat after me: "Biological food cravings are normal. When I fulfill them, I'm caring for myself." And forget all about weight-loss diets.

■ WHY DIETS FAIL ■

With the majority of Americans on a diet at any given moment, I'll make an assumption. At some point in your life, you've restricted calories.

Maybe you lost excess pounds and have kept them off. If so, great. More than likely, you regained all or some of the weight.

Do you know the reason for your regained pounds? Cravings, pure and simple.

At a physiological level, your body behaves as it did millions of years ago. When you diet, it thinks you might become a victim of a life-threatening famine and will fight hard to hold on to fat, even if you've got more than your fair share. To get you to eat, your body will release neuropeptide Y and galanin, along with other body chemicals.

Truly, you've never failed on a diet. The diet failed you.

The typical diet restricts calories and works against your natural and normal biological food cravings. Even if you possess amazing willpower, you're bound to trip up eventually. Any diet "failure" is a testimony to the power of neurotransmitters.

Your neurotransmitters are powerful indeed. They can clear your thinking or make it dim, enhance your mood or bust it, and—of course—propel your body to peak physical performance. And how.

■ THE COMMONSENSE CRAVER'S CUSTOMIZER ■

Before we get to the specifics, a few words: Biological food cravings are normal and natural. They tell you what your body needs
for optimal functioning. They open the door to the "Aha!" experience that gets you on an exhilarating mental-emotional-
physical roll. So listen to your biological food cravings and satisfy
them.

As mentioned, a biological food craving differs from an emotional food craving. The latter accompanies negative feelings,
such as loneliness, anger, upset, or boredom, and you eat to feel
better. The problem is, any good feelings are short-lived, and you
often have to deal with the resulting guilt and self-deprecation
caused by your perceived weakness. In contrast, a biological craving is brought on by changes in your brain chemistry. If your
craving is for a specific food, it doesn't diminish over time, and
it can be satisfied with a small amount, it's most likely biological.

1. *Eat the commonsense craver's foods.*

Any food for which you have a *biological* craving—whether
for french fries, Ding Dongs, broccoli, or, yes, prime rib—is legitimate and you need to fulfill the craving for optimal functioning.

Any food for which you have an *emotional* craving should
not be fulfilled because it'll make you think, feel, and perform
poorly. Rather, you need to identify the emotion prompting the
craving and deal with the emotion. For example, if you're angry,
write your thoughts in a journal or exercise to release pent-up
frustration.

Unlike biological cravings, the emotional ones usually pass in
ten to thirty minutes.

2. *Eat the commonsense craver's foods at the right times.*

The right time to satisfy a *biological* craving is within a few
minutes. If you try to outlast it, the craving will get stronger while
your mood worsens, and you're more likely to overeat.

There is never a right time to give in to an *emotional* craving. Though eating to satisfy a biological craving enhances your mood, emotional eating makes you feel worse.

3. Eat the commonsense craver's foods in the right combos.

The right combo for a *biological* craving is whatever your body desires but in small amounts. You can also use some clues to figure out what you need. Are you mentally sluggish? Is your concentration poor? Do you feel tired? If the answer to any of these is yes, then you'll probably have a hankering for protein, such as cheese, skim milk, or legumes. Are you nervous, stressed-out, or feeling sad? You'll probably desire carbos, including sweets like ice cream and doughnuts and starches like whole-grain muffins and rice pilaf.

As you've figured out by now, there is no right food combo for an *emotional* craving. The combo that makes sense is exercising, having a strong support network, and understanding why you eat to "stuff" emotions, with the help of a professional if necessary.

Commonsense craver's tip of the day: When your body says eat, eat.

Pumping Up Your Body Power

One of the earliest historical accounts of the physical advantages of power-eating spotlights a teen, his buddies, and a king. The king insists they eat the rich, meaty delicacies from his royal table. The teens refuse. They go veg instead.

The place: Babylon.

The year: about 605 B.C.

The main players: Nebuchadnezzar, king of Babylon, and Daniel, an outspoken, handsome teenager and Israelite who had been taken captive along with three of his friends. The teens are being groomed for service in the king's palace.

Let's listen in.

The king of Babylon ordered the chief of his court officials to bring in some of the Israelites—young men without any physical defect, handsome, showing aptitude for every kind of learning, and qualified to serve in the king's palace. The king assigned them a daily amount of food and wine from the king's table.

But Daniel resolved not to defile himself with the royal food and wine, and he asked the chief official for permission [to eat vegetables and water only]. The official told Daniel, "I am afraid of my lord the king, who has assigned your food and drink. Why should he see you looking worse than

*the other young men your age? The king would then have
my head because of you."*

*Daniel then said to the guard whom the chief official had
appointed over Daniel, Hananiah, Mishael, and Azariah,
"Please test your servants for ten days: Give us nothing but
vegetables to eat and water to drink. Then compare our appearance with that of the young men who eat the royal
food." So the guard agreed to this and tested them for ten
days.*

*At the end of the ten days, they looked healthier and
better nourished than any of the young men who ate the
royal food. So the guard took away their choice food and
the wine they were to drink and gave them vegetables instead.*

*At the end of the time set by the king to bring them, the
chief official presented them to Nebuchadnezzar. The king
talked with them, and he found none equal to Daniel, Hananiah, Mishael, and Azariah; so they entered the king's service.*

Daniel 1:3–19 (New International Version)

The king found none—not one—equal to Daniel and his
friends. They looked strong and healthy; they were energetic,
smart, and contented; they were, in the king's opinion, perfect
models of all a man ought to be.

And little did the king know that Daniel and his friends had
forsaken the royal food for ordinary vegetables and water!

▪ WHAT EXACTLY IS BODY POWER? ▪

Think back to the last time you felt strong, agile, quick and fo-
cused, bursting with energy. Perhaps you experienced the delightful sense of physical mastery during yesterday's tennis set or last
week's gym workout. Or must your mind travel to your youth
for an example of body power?

Though I experience body power today, my favorite expression of strength, energy, and stamina dates to my childhood. With blond pigtails and a quiet demeanor, I looked the part of a pint-sized damsel in distress, but I was a tomboy at heart. I loved to jump fences, climb tall trees, stomp in rain puddles, and challenge boys to running races. I learned early on the freedom that comes with strength and stamina.

But you know how it goes. As we age, many of us prefer the sidelines to the action. We declare an end to our climbing and jumping days. If we do dare to be active, we too often find comfort on a NordicTrack while watching CNN.

Here's the good news: You can reclaim and enhance body power. Just be reasonable.

For instance, as a kid, I flip-flopped my tawny body around the backyard. No way will I attempt difficult gymnastic maneuvers today. My thirty-seven-year-old frame prefers fitness walks, weight-lifting, dancing with my girls to Raffi and the Beach Boys, and, I confess, an occasional climb in the branches of a spreading maple tree.

Body power has a two-part definition. Without one or the other, you're falling short of your true potential.

I've mentioned the first part, the components of physical well-being: strength, energy, endurance, agility, fast reaction time, and balance. This is your outer expression of body power.

Your inner expression of body power is equally important:

- Blood pressure of 120/80 is considered an optimal reading. A little lower if you're in good health is fine too. If your blood pressure is consistently above 140/90, there is cause for concern.
- Total cholesterol of about 150 mg/dL.
- High-density lipoprotein (the "good" cholesterol) at greater than 35 mg/dL.
- Blood triglyceride levels at less than 250 mg/dL.
- Normal blood glucose level.
- A healthy weight and ratio of lean and fat tissues.

- Any other sign that your health practitioner has deemed important for you.

You might wonder why I listed "healthy weight" under the inner expression of body power. Simple. Though you can see whether a person appears too fat or too skinny, the damage of malnutrition (with obesity as our culture's prime example) takes its greatest toll on the inner workings of the body, leading to a cascade of illnesses: heart disease, stroke, some cancers, adult-onset diabetes, to name some of them.

To repeat, a superfit body has the strength, energy, and stamina for work and play, exercise and physical competition. It has measurable signs of health and is able to resist and withstand disease at every stage of life—yesterday, today, and as many tommorows that have been written for you.

■ TWO WAYS TO ACHIEVE BODY POWER ■

Just as there are two parts to the definition of body power, interdependent gateways lead to its achievement.

The first gateway: the power-eating promise. When you power-eat, you give your body the food it needs to function at its best. I'm talking protein, fat, and carbohydrates, the three macronutrients—"macro" meaning large, because your body needs them in relatively large amounts—eaten in a proper mix. You'll discover the healthiest mix for you in a moment.

Curiously, many active people have their nutrition all wrong. They often think the prescription for a healthy meal is loading up on protein (like Rocky Balboa and his infamous raw egg concoction). They eat too much fat and protein—and the wrong types of protein—and not enough carbos. Remember, protein doesn't make muscle. Exercise does.

The second gateway: exercise. Remember the saying "use it or lose it"? It holds true with body power. When you are actively "using it," you won't lose—and can gain—your strength, stamina, energy, or any of the other hallmarks of body power. Sorry, super-glued couch potatoes, but you must get up and go reclaim the vigor of your youth to achieve body power.

Answer these questions and find out whether you know sports nutrition basics:

1. You need to eat about 30 percent of your total calories from fat to achieve optimal physical performance. *True False*
2. Many vegetarians barely meet their protein requirements. *True False*
3. Eggs are the best source of protein. *True False*
4. When you want to lose weight, body fat is the best fuel to burn. *True False*
5. Eating the right foods to manufacture certain neurotransmitters is the key to body power. *True False*

DRINK UP

What happens when you forget to water the houseplants? They droop. The same goes for you when you drink too little water.

Many people walk around feeling sluggish or "off" and don't realize why. Research shows that even slight dehydration can zap your energy and ruin your mood. Your body's cells contain countless chemicals and nutrients, and they function best when they're diluted in just the right amount of fluid.

Don't rely on your body's thirst mechanism to tell you when to down a glass or two of water. It may not kick in until moderate dehydration is setting in. Rather, sip the equivalent of six to eight eight-ounce glasses of fluids throughout the day.

The fluids can be water, juice, and broth, but not alcohol or caffeinated beverages, both of which are diuretics. Drink even more water during hot weather or when you exercise, about two eight-ounce glasses per pound of weight lost.

As you increase your water intake, you'll notice other changes beyond stepped-up energy: more frequent urination and light-colored urine.

In fact, a telltale sign that you're drinking a healthy amount of water is the color and smell of your urine. Not good: dark yellow and a mineral odor. Very good: light yellow or clear and no odor.

Enough bathroom talk.

If you chose *false* for each of the above questions, you're right on the mark. Here are brief explanations, which I'll expand in this chapter and the next.

Misconception: You need to eat about 30 percent of total calories from fat to achieve optimal physical performance. Various health organizations have tossed around "30 percent" as a goal for all Americans to achieve. But the ideal is 20 to 25 percent, most of the top nutrition experts agree. Many ultra athletes inch their fat intake even lower.

Misconception: Many vegetarians barely meet their protein requirements. The truth is, many vegetarians take in double the amount of protein that their bodies actually require. Research confirms that vegetarians who eat sufficient calories from a variety of foods do not have protein shortfalls. (See "The Truth About Protein," page 14.)

Misconception: Eggs are the best source of protein. For rats, yes. For people, no. The egg was once considered the "perfect" protein, but the studies pointing to this conclusion relied on rats, not people, for their data. People thrive on such protein sources as soy foods, legumes, and certain higher-protein grains—and, if you choose to include them, low-fat and nonfat dairy products and, yes, an occasional omelet.

Misconception: When you want to lose weight, body fat is the best fuel to burn. Your cleanest burning fuel is carbos, stored as glycogen in your muscles and liver. To lose weight, you need to burn a carbo-fat mixture—not fat alone. This is one reason why a low-carbo diet is a poor choice; your body needs adequate carbos to function at its best.

Misconception: Eating the right foods to manufacture certain neurotransmitters is the key to body power. Gotcha! With brain power and mood power, neurotransmitters are a driving force, as you discovered in the previous chapters, but they take a backseat when we talk body power. They still play a role in getting you in the groove to eat right and exercise, but their influence is indirect.

Picture the indirect influence as a circle.

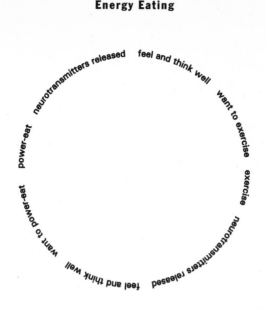

A side note: The endorphins do count in exercise. But it's in "hitting the wall," as marathoners put it, that these neurotransmitters are released. Luckily, you can get an endorphin rush without running yourself into the ground. In chapter 8 I'll show you how.

■ THE BEST MIX FOR YOU ■

To achieve the power-eating promise, you need a healthy balance of neurotransmitters *and* a healthy mix of the three macronutrients: protein, fat, and carbos. Balancing your neurotransmitters and eating a healthy mix of foods go hand in hand: When you overeat or undereat any one of the three macronutrients, your brain chemistry will be "off" (i.e., unbalanced). And, because your neurotransmitters determine how well you think, feel, and function, you'll experience the suboptimal consequences of overall malaise.

What is the healthiest mix of macronutrients?

In general, most of the top nutrition experts agree that the best mix of protein, fat, and carbos is this:

10 to 15 percent protein
20 to 25 percent fat
60 to 70 percent carbos

These are percentages of total calories in the overall diet and need not dictate a single meal or a day of meals. Talk of percentages can get boring fast. So let's put your face on the numbers.

Suppose you're a forty-year-old woman (plus or minus a few years) in generally good health. Your height and weight are about average, though like most Americans you'd like better tone to show off in your swimsuit. You're moderately active—neither a triathlete nor sedentary.

Your total caloric requirements would be about 2,000 a day. For your diet to fall in the experts' ranges, you'd need 200 to 300 protein calories, 400 to 500 fat calories, and 1,200 to 1,400 carbohydrate calories daily.

Let's make the numbers easier to use by converting them into grams. Remember, protein and carbohydrates have four calories per gram, while fat is twice as "expensive," with nine calories per gram.

Thus your daily diet would consist of 50 to 75 grams of protein, 44 to 56 grams of fat, and 300 to 350 grams of carbos. Going another step, let's look at a typical day's meals and snacks that fit these numbers.

BREAKFAST	SNACK	LUNCH	SNACK	DINNER
Whole-grain cereal with milk; orange juice; tea	Yogurt and fruit; spritzer	Bean burrito with cheese, tomatoes, lettuce, and sour cream; rice; iced tea	Bagel with cream cheese; milk	Vegetable lasagna; glazed carrots; salad; crusty bread; chocolate mousse

Equally important, the day's meals and snacks must satisfy your need for delicious food. As I've said before, if the food doesn't tickle your taste buds, why eat it? (Be sure to check out the recipes in part 3.)

You've seen the big picture. Now the details.

■ GETTING TOO MUCH PROTEIN? ■

Guess how many grams of protein the typical vegetarian gobbles up in a day. For a man, 105 grams; for a woman, 65 grams. (Even the average vegan, who eats no animal foods, not even cheese, milk, or eggs, gets ample protein.) A person who regularly eats meat? For a man, 103 grams; for a woman, 74 grams.

Now compare these numbers to the Recommended Dietary Allowance (RDA). For women aged nineteen and over (at 120 pounds), protein needs are 44 grams daily. The RDA for their male counterparts (at 154 pounds) is 56 grams of protein daily.

It's a no-brainer: The typical vegetarian eats ample protein— arguably too much protein in some cases—while meat-eaters take in two to three times the RDA and far above the recommendations of most nutrition experts.

Getting adequate protein is important, for it performs many crucial functions. Protein builds and rebuilds tissues, including muscle, aids your immune system, helps carry nutrients throughout the body, and helps form hormones and enzymes.

But when you take in too much protein, your body must work overtime to get rid of it. Protein is never used for energy, unless you're starving. In that case, after exhausting your stores of carbos and fat, your body will ravage your muscles for food to keep you functioning. Not a pretty sight.

Though excess protein can be converted to body fat or stored as carbos, your body normally gets rid of it. During the taking apart of amino acids, the nitrogen part is freed. Excess nitrogen in your system is poisonous. It must be detoxified. In the process, ammonia, another toxin, is created. Eventually it is turned into urea and excreted via the kidneys, taxing them.

Susceptible people with protein overload may experience kidney problems, even cancer. In one study, researchers analyzed the diets of 690 kidney cancer patients and found that people who ate a lot of meat, eggs, milk, cheese, and, surprisingly, cereals, were 90 percent more likely to suffer kidney tumors than those who ate modest amounts of protein.

The upshot: Take in a healthy amount of protein. But don't eat too much of it. It may spell disease.

That said, let's talk about you.

You've heard the RDAs for the typical woman and man. But what are your specific protein needs? To find out, consider these questions.

How much do you weigh? What's your regular physical activity? Are you pregnant or lactating? Do you have a chronic illness? Your answers will add up to your individual protein needs.

If you're sedentary, the RDA for protein is 0.36

COUNT ON PROTEIN

Chances are, you're getting ample protein even if you exercise or train for competition every day.

A moderately active person who works out almost every day at fairly high intensity needs about 0.5 to 0.7 grams of protein per pound of body weight each day. This translates to 60 to 84 grams for a 120-pound person, and 80 to 112 grams for a 160-pound person. Wonderfully, you'll get more protein as you step up your exercise, simply because you'll eat more to maintain your weight.

Here are some foods listed with their protein contents in grams.

GRAINS

Barley, whole grain (½ cup cooked): 3g
Buckwheat, whole grain (½ cup cooked): 3.5g
Bulgur (½ cup cooked): 5g
Cornmeal (¼ cup): 4g
Millet, whole grain (½ cup cooked): 1.5g
Rice, brown (½ cup cooked): 2.5g
Rolled oats (½ cup cooked): 3g
Soybean flour, defatted (¼ cup): 12g
Wheat berries (hard red winter, ½ cup cooked): 4g
Wheat flour
  all-purpose (¼ cup): 2.5g
  whole (¼ cup): 4g
  bread (whole wheat, 1 slice): 4g
Wheat germ, toasted (2 tablespoons): 4g

VEGETABLES

Artichoke (1 medium cooked): 3.5g
Asparagus (⅔ cup cooked): 3g
Beets (sliced, ½ cup cooked): 1g
Green beans (½ cup cooked): 1g
Green peas (½ cup cooked): 1.5g
Greens (beet, collard, dandelion, mustard, turnip, ½ cup cooked): 2–3g
Broccoli (½ cup cooked): 2.5g
Brussels sprouts (½ cup cooked): 2.5g
Carrot (1 medium, raw): 1g
Cauliflower (½ cup cooked): 1g
Corn (kernels, ½ cup cooked): 3g

Eggplant (½ cup diced): 1g
Kale (½ cup cooked): 2.5g
Okra (½ cup cooked): 1.5g
Potato (1 medium, baked): 4g
Spinach (1 cup, raw): 1.5g
Tomato (1 medium, raw): 1g
Turnip (½ cup cooked): 0.5g

FRUITS

All types (½ cup or 1 medium): trace to 1.5g

NUTS & SEEDS

All types (2 tablespoons): 2–3g
Nut butters (2 tablespoons): 5–8g

LEGUMES

Black beans (½ cup cooked): 6g
Black-eyed peas (½ cup cooked): 6g
Chickpeas (½ cup cooked): 7g
Great northern beans (½ cup cooked): 7g
Kidney beans (½ cup cooked): 7.5g
Lentils (½ cup cooked): 7.5g
Lima beans (½ cup cooked): 8g
Pinto beans (½ cup cooked): 7.5g
Soybeans (½ cup cooked): 10g
Split peas (½ cup cooked): 8g
Tempeh (2 ounces): 11g
Tofu (½ cup, firm, raw): 20g

DAIRY PRODUCTS

Cheese (1 ounce): 6–8g
Cottage cheese, low-fat (½ cup): 16g
Ice cream (½ cup): 2g
Milk, nonfat (1 cup): 8g
Yogurt, low-fat (1 cup): 13g

EGGS & MEAT

Egg
  whole: 6g
  white only: 3g
  yolk only: 3g
Meat, all types (3 ounces): about 25g

FATS & SWEETS

All types: trace

grams per pound of body weight. To calculate your protein requirement, multiply your weight by 0.36 grams:

0.36 grams × your weight in pounds = the number of protein grams you need per day

For example, if you weigh 150 pounds, multiply 150 by 0.36 and you will find that you require 54 grams of protein per day.

But you're active, right? At least I hope so. Exercise is crucial to your achieving the power-eating promise. For active people, protein needs vary according to the type of exercise and the intensity of the exercise.

Strength-training. If you lift weights, work out on Nautilus or similar machines, use specially designed rubber bands that create resistance, or take part in a strength sport like the clean-and-jerk, you need about 0.7 grams of protein per pound of body weight. This assumes you strength-train regularly (three to five times weekly) with moderate to high intensity. If you strength-train less than three times a week with low to moderate intensity, your protein needs are between 0.36 grams and 0.7 grams of protein per pound of body weight.

Strength-trainers can use this equation to figure protein needs:

0.7 grams × your weight in pounds = the number of protein grams you need each day

As you'll learn in chapter 8, the American College of Sports Medicine recommends strength-training for just about everyone. For instance, in building muscle, you increase your lean tissue mass, which, in turn, boosts your metabolism. Your risk of osteoporosis lessens too. Another bonus: You look and feel younger, stronger, and more energetic.

Aerobics. If you do heart-strengthening aerobics—from jogging and fitness walks to dancing and cycling—you need about 0.5 grams of protein per pound of body weight. This assumes you do aerobics regularly (three to five times weekly) with moderate to high intesity. If you jog, walk, dance, or the like less than three times a week and with low to moderate intensity, your protein needs are between 0.36 grams and 0.5 grams of protein per pound of body weight.

Aerobics aficionados can use this equation to figure protein needs:

0.5 grams × your weight in pounds = the number of protein grams you need each day

Cross-training. Cross-training is exactly what it sounds like: a mix of aerobics and strength-training. Some cross-trainers combine the two in a single sport like rugby, which requires both strength and stamina. Others go a step farther, pairing a strength-training sport like weight-lifting with beach volleyball, Rollerblading, or dancing.

Cross-trainers may need as much as 0.9 grams of protein per pound of body weight if—and this is a big "if"—they work intensely at their endurance and strength exercises and sports. Most of us who play tennis or soccer once a week, hit the weights at the gym occasionally, and stroll our toddlers now and then need far less than 0.9 grams of protein per pound of body weight. We could probably get by on half that figure.

Serious cross-trainers, here's the math to figure your protein needs:

0.9 grams × your weight in pounds = the number of protein grams you need each day

As I'm sure you've noticed, your protein needs do increase when you're active. But you probably are getting ample protein already. Remember, the typical vegetarian and almost vegetarian easily exceed the RDA. If you're curious to find out your protein intake, simply record the foods you eat in what amounts for at least three days. A week is better. Then count your protein grams. (See "Count on Protein," page 114, for common foods and their protein content.)

▪ THE RIGHT FATS ▪

The less fat you eat, the better. Right?

Not necessarily.

I hedge for three reasons: First, your body requires fat in the diet, but only a tiny amount of the essential fatty acids linoleic acid, which must be obtained from food or supplements. (See sidebar, "Getting Enough Omega-3s?") Second, as mentioned, some fats are better for you than others. The worst are saturated fats and trans fatty acids. The good fats are monounsaturates, like olive oil and canola oil.

Third, fat adds flavor to food. Banning it from the kitchen is a culinary mistake—and a healthy lifestyle snafu.

If you choose a spartan diet, your neurotransmitters rebel.

They barrage your brain with messages to eat, eat, eat. Usually they call out for fat and sugar when they think they're facing starvation. Fat and sugar in excess wipes out body power as well as brain power and mood power.

That's why I recommend a moderate amount of fat in the diet. Your neurotransmitters are happy, your food tastes great, and your risk of diet-related illnesses plummets. A win-win-win combo.

As mentioned, a health-smart percentage of total calories from fat is 20 to 25 percent. Most of the top nutrition experts favor this range because it fuels up your body in the best way, giving you the strength and stamina for work and play, exercise and physical competition, and reducing your risk of chronic illness and their signs, like high blood pressure.

Your fat should come mostly from unsaturated types—monounsaturates and polyunsaturates. Assuming a 20 percent fat diet, aim for 8 percent monounsaturated

---

GETTING ENOUGH OMEGA-3s?

Fish sales leaped out of the culinary waters after several research studies linked the omega-3 fatty acids in fish and shellfish to the prevention of heart disease. Then the health-conscious learned of seafood contamination.

The U.S. Food and Drug Administration (FDA) reports that cases of food poisoning from seafood number about 113,000 each year. This is clearly an underestimation, because many cases go unreported.

A solution: safe vegetarian sources of omega-3s.

Alpha-linolenic acid (LNA), a stellar omega-3, is found in plant foods. The body can convert it to two other types of omega 3s, docosahexenoic acid (DHA) and eicosapentenoic acid (EPA). These omega-3s all help control blood clotting.

In 1996, the American Heart Association stated in an advisory that tofu, soybean oil, canola oil, wheat germ, butternuts (also called "white walnuts"), and walnuts are important sources of LNA. In addition, flaxseed oil, flax seeds, and purslane, an herb that's part of the traditional Mediterranean diet, contain healthy amounts of linolenic acid.

You need not eat extra fat to get LNA. Simply use LNA-rich foods in your usual diet. For instance, sauté vegetables in canola oil, sprinkle wheat germ on breakfast cereal, and add purslane and a few teaspoons of walnuts to a salad.

Linoleic acid is another essential fatty acid that must be obtained from the foods you eat. Rich sources are safflower oil, nuts, and wheat germ. Some researchers believe that a healthy vegetarian diet, which is naturally high in linoleic acid and low in arachidonic acid, protects against cancer.

fat, 7 percent polyunsaturated fat, and only 5 percent saturated fat.

Here's the math:

Step 1: Figure the ideal total fat intake for you:

your total daily calories × *0.20 (or 0.25)* = *calories from fat*

Now divide this figure by 9 (because there are nine calories in a gram of fat):

calories from fat ÷ *9* = *grams of total fat*

Step 2: Figure the highest number of grams of saturated fats you may have:

your total daily calories × *0.5* = *calories from saturated fats*
÷ 9 = _____ *grams of saturated fats*

Knowing these numbers will help you eat a fat-favorable diet and achieve peak physical performance, as will fueling up on carbos.

▪ THE BODY POWER GIANT ▪

Of the three macronutrients, carbos write your meal ticket to peak physical performance. They are your body's number-one source of energy—energy to hike the Appalachian trail, to open a jar of pickles, to lift a toddler, to play a game of squash.

Suppose it's time for your strength-training workout. Short bursts of effort, as you complete a set of biceps curls or leg presses, for instance, require a fuel mix of 95 percent carbos and 5 percent fat.

These numbers change dramatically when you aerobicize. During aerobic exercise, your body burns mostly carbos at first, gobbling up glucose circulating in the blood. As you keep on exercising at a mild to moderate pace, your heart pumps harder and more blood flows into your tissues. Now fat can be burned too, because oxygen must be present in the cells. The fuel mix will be about half carbos, half fat. Eventually, your body reverts to burning up stored carbos. The more carbos you have stored as glycogen, the longer you stay active and increase your strength and endurance.

Carbos not only energize you but also are the key for building lean mass—in other words, muscle. And the more muscle you have, the less flab you put on.

That's because muscle uses more energy, even if you're snoozing, than do other body tissues except the brain. Your metabolism (the rate at which you burn calories) goes up when you've got more muscle.

But back to the key point: To make muscles, load your plate with carbos and exercise.

Don't get me wrong. Protein is essential too. In fact, studies have shown some interesting results when people meet their protein needs. For instance, researchers at Kent State

---

DO ENERGY BARS WORK?

Yes. Should you spend your money on them? Probably not.

Whether you call them energy bars, sports bars, nutrition bars, or glorified candy bars, these high-priced confections are no substitute for power-eating. For peak physical performance, you need to eat right (lots of carbos, moderate fat, adequate protein, and ample nutrients), plenty of water and exercise, or training, specific to your needs.

Energy bars deliver calories, with more from protein and less from fat than a Snickers. They are fortified with nutrients, too.

But the best sources of energy are complex carbos (starches) packaged in food, not wrappers. Complex carbos are broken down into blood glucose during digestion. Some glucose is used immediately for energy. The rest is stored as glycogen in the muscles and liver (or converted to fat if you eat more food than your body needs). When you need energy, the body uses a mix of glycogen and fat to power muscles. Without a doubt, complex carbos reign as the main fuel for your body, especially your muscles and brain.

Most energy bars, however, list among their ingredients such simple carbos (sugars) as high fructose corn syrup, honey, fructose, high maltose corn syrup, and dextrose. The sugar may give you a temporary energy boost as your blood glucose rises, but you may feel depleted in an hour or so.

Your best bet: Eat a real meal, not an energy bar, except in the very few instances (I hope) that you only have time for the quickest snack. Energy bars are better than candy and they're better than nothing. Just don't buy into the energy-bar-as-food hype.

University divided people in its study into three groups of avid strength trainers: the first group followed a lower protein diet, the second followed a moderate protein diet (about 0.6 grams per pound of body weight), and the third followed a higher protein diet (about 1 gram per pound of body weight).

Interestingly, increasing protein intake to 0.6 grams triggered protein synthesis, an indicator of muscle growth, but upping protein intake from 0.6 grams to 1 gram didn't cause more protein synthesis. The lower protein group (about 0.4 grams per pound of body weight) showed no protein synthesis.

The bottom line: To achieve body power, meet your individual protein needs (which you determined using the equations on pages 115–117) *and* load up on carbos.

■ A PLATEFUL OF PHYTOCHEMICALS ■

May I suggest a lunch of romaine topped with mounds of shredded carrot, red cabbage, sliced onion, chopped broccoli, and legumes and tossed in a light dressing of balsamic vinegar, garlic, and soybean oil? This meal supplies much more than vitamins, minerals, and fiber. It's got phytochemicals, lots of them.

Phytochemicals means "plant chemicals." They're found mostly in carbo-rich foods, which is good news for power-eaters. When you follow the Power-Up Food Plan (chapter 7), your body is getting plenty of phytochemicals. In the long run, taking in adequate phytochemicals may help protect against disease. In the short run, some phytochemicals work with other body chemicals to give you energy.

There are thousands of phytochemicals. Here are descriptions of a few of them:

Carotenoids. Found in orange and yellow fruits and vegetables, carotenoids may prevent damage to cell membranes and the genetic material inside cells.

Genistein. Found in soybeans and its derivatives (tofu, tempeh, soymilk, and so on), genistein reduces blood cholesterol levels.

Indoles. Found in broccoli, cauliflower, cabbage, and Brussels sprouts, indoles help reduce estrogen, thereby possibly reducing breast cancer risk.

Lycopene. Found in tomatoes, lycopene may help protect against heart disease and cancer.

Tannins. Found in tea, tannins lower blood pressure and reduce blood cholesterol.

And that's only a taste. The thousands of phytochemicals in delicious vegetarian cuisine power up the inner workings of your body. They help keep you free from illness and give you vigor. It's a culinary bonanza: Eat right and you're well on your way to peak physical performance.

■ THEN WHY EXERCISE? ■

You might think, "If following the Power-Up Food Plan gives me body power, why not just power-eat to my heart's content and skip regular exercise?"

See if you can recall why the experts are high on exercise. Choose among the following:

1. Exercise revs up your metabolism, which helps you maintain a healthy weight.
2. Exercise can trigger the release of the endorphins, the feel-good neurotransmitters that puts you in the mood for more exercise.
3. Research shows inactivity is as dangerous to your health as a smoking habit.

Well, the right answer is all three. Power-eating, when combined with exercise (both aerobic and strength-training), gives you strength, energy, stamina, and agility as well as enviable inner signs of body power, including healthy blood pressure, cholesterol, blood sugar, and weight.

Achieving peak physical performance doesn't stop at the here and now. It can be yours for a lifetime.

■ THE SUPER-FIT CUSTOMIZER ■

To achieve peak physical performance, you must give your body plenty of carbos, adequate protein for your sport, and enough but not too much fat in addition to health-promoting phytochemicals and lots of fluids. The core of the Power-Up Food Plan satisfies the weekend athlete, but for super fitness, pay attention to the following guidelines.

1. *Eat super-fit foods.* Here are examples.

CARBOS	PROTEIN	FAT
Complex carbos, such as whole grains, vegetables, fruits	Lean protein, such as legumes, including soy foods, low-fat dairy products, egg whites, and high-protein grains	Mono- and unsaturated fats up to 25 percent of total daily caloric intake
Limit simple carbos, such as candy, cakes, and pies		

Also drink a minimum of six eight-ounce glasses of water plus two more eight-ounce glasses of water per every pound lost during exercise.

2. *Eat super-fit foods at the right times.*

To get adequate calories, you'll need to eat many meals— some will be nutrient-dense snacks—throughout the day. Be sure to eat a small meal no sooner than one hour before your workout or competition. By eating ahead, your food will have time to digest, at least partially, so you won't feel weighed down.

3. *Eat super-fit foods in the right combos.*

While the protein-for-alertness and carbos-only-for-calm principles hold true for peak performance, your best combo most of the time will be a protein-carbo mix. Carbos are of utmost importance because the body uses them for fuel, so no skimping. You need protein too. It's crucial to the body in many ways, including keeping your energy up. However, whenever you feel tense or blue, choose carbos only. The resulting increase in your brain serotonin levels will help calm you.

Super-fit tip of the day: Everyone can achieve peak performance through power-eating and physical activity.

POWER QUIZ

How Fit Are Your Choices?

Many active people have their nutrition all wrong. They may believe any number of myths: that eating protein builds muscles; that an energy bar is a nutritious meal; that higher-fat meals are fine as long as you're active. To see if you make body-smart decisions, answer these questions.

1. Which best describes your typical breakfast?

    a) two waffles with syrup and coffee
    b) a big bowl of bran cereal with skim milk, fruit, and a glass of water
    c) scrambled eggs, toast, and juice
    d) coffee and a danish

2. Which best describes your typical lunch?

    a) linguine with marinara sauce, garlic bread, and frozen yogurt
    b) black bean chili with corn bread, a vegetable salad, and juice
    c) a peanut butter and jelly sandwich, potato chips, an apple, and a soda
    d) a piece of fruit

3. Which best describes your typical dinner?

   a) a vegetable sauté over brown rice, coffee, and a brownie
   b) pasta primavera in a light cheese sauce, garlic bread, fruit, and a glass of water
   c) grilled chicken, mashed potatoes, green beans, and a glass of wine
   d) a slice of pizza

4. Which best describes your typical snack?

   a) a sweet, like cookies
   b) whole-wheat crackers with fruit spread
   c) potato chips
   d) nothing

5. Rate your typical energy level.

   a) low   b) high   c) moderate

6. Rate your typical reaction time.

   a) low   b) high   c) moderate

7. Rate your typical agility.

   a) not very agile   b) definitely agile
   c) somewhat agile

8. Rate your typical endurance.

   a) poor   b) great   c) okay

9. Rate your typical strength.

   a) poor   b) great   c) okay

10. Which best describes your workout pattern?

    a) aerobic exercise three times a week for about thirty minutes per session
    b) a combination of aerobic exercise, strength-training, and gentle stretching three to five times a week for about thirty minutes per session
    c) strength-training six days a week for an hour per session
    d) no particular pattern—just occasional workouts

11. How much nonalcoholic fluid do you drink after working out?

    a) a cup of water or juice per every pound of water weight lost during exercise
    b) two cups of water or juice per every pound of water weight lost during exercise
    c) about a liter of pop
    d) as much water as necessary to no longer feel thirsty

12. Which do you believe is the best fuel for working muscles?

    a) simple carbohydrates   b) complex carbohydrates
    c) protein and carbohydrates d) fiber

13. How often do you eat iron-rich foods, like legumes and dried fruits, preferably with a food high in vitamin C?

    a) several times a week   b) every day
    c) rarely   d) once or twice a week

14. How often do you eat foods rich in phytochemicals?

    a) several times a day   b) at every meal and snack
    c) occasionally

15. Do you eat enough calories to meet the higher energy needs of an active person?

   a) usually   b) always
   c) occasionally

   _____

   Give yourself a point for every b answer and tally your score. The highest possible score is 15.

   12 to 15: Excellent! Your food and exercise choices show that you're treating your body well.

   8 to 11: Okay, but making better body-wise choices will mean greater gains in energy, strength, and other hallmarks of body power.

   Less than 8: Shape up your choices now. Until you do, body power will be as elusive as Barry Sanders on the football field.

Living Longer,
Living Better

Japanese parents tell this fable to their children: Long, long ago, a young man named Urashima lived in a village on the coast. He was wise and kind beyond his years. Some say he was a handsome prince; others say he was a master fisherman.

One day Urashima walked the beach and saw a group of mean-spirited children pounding a gigantic turtle with sticks. His heart was filled with compassion for the turtle, and he rescued it. The turtle thanked him by inviting him to travel with it, far beneath the blue-green waves, to a palace of coral.

Here, in the Turtle's Paradise, as it's called, life is enchanted, filled with joy and music and friends and food. No one sheds a tear. No one feels pain or gets sick. And no one ever grows old.

Researchers say a place like the Turtle's Paradise really exists on our planet. It is Okinawa, a cluster of islands four hundred miles southwest of Japan.

Okinawa boasts a large number of centenarians, with certified documents to prove their birthdays. What's more, they remain remarkably healthy into their eighties, nineties, and hundreds. The reason for Okinawans' "body power" seems to have less to do with their genetics than with their diet and lifestyle. Studies report that Okinawans who move to mainland Japan or California and adopt the eating and living habits of their new homes experience shortened life and more illnesses.

So what's the Okinawans' secret to longevity and well-being? I count at least three:

• power-eating
• activity and exercise
• close ties to family and friends

As mentioned in the previous chapter, body power has a two-part, mutually inclusive definition. If you fall short in one or the other, peak physical performance is out of reach.

In the previous chapter we discussed the basics for achieving the first part of the definition: body power as strength, endurance, energy, agility, balance, and quick reaction time. Body power is a delightful sense of physical mastery. It is the optimal level of health your body is genetically programmed to achieve when given the chance. Like other power-eaters, you become less prone to chronic illness like heart disease and cancer and can significantly increase your odds of living long and living well—in other words, experiencing your own personal Turtle's Paradise.

Here we illuminate the second part of the body-power definition: living long and living well.

■ STRETCHING YOUR YEARS ■

American women live an average of seventy-nine years, inching out American men by seven years. The Okinawans, as you may have guessed, fare better. The men live nearly seventy-six years (that's four years longer than American men), and the women, an impressive eighty-four-plus years. No other region of Japan, or the world for that matter (unless you count the Republic of Georgia, south of Russia, where scientists suspect age is routinely exaggerated), enjoys greater longevity.

The Okinawans are almost vegetarian. Their bowls are piled high with rice, root vegetables, leafy greens, soy foods (like tofu), fish, and, believe it or not, bits of pork. Pork, in fact, is considered a national treasure, an import from China six centuries ago that never left. It's used to flavor soups, noodle dishes, just about everything.

And yet carbos make up the bulk of the Okinawans' diet, followed by fat (at about 25 percent of total calories, significantly lower than Americans' 34 percent average) then protein. Their diet is low in processed foods and sugar, and rich in fiber, thanks to their love of vegetables and grains. And they eat modestly; few Okinawans are obese.

American vegetarians, too, bask in the light of greater longevity than do people who eat meat regularly. Research shows that male vegetarians live an average of about nine years longer than their nonvegetarian counterparts, and women seven and a half years longer.

When you analyze these numbers, it's clear: American vegetarians enjoy longer life than the longest living people on Earth—the Okinawans!

So unpack your Okinawa-destined suitcases and stay awhile. Vegetarians and

---

MORE SATISFYING SEX

Some lovers say champagne gets them in the mood. Others favor artichokes, chocolate, or any number of taste treats. While food lore identifies culinary aphrodisiacs, the most overlooked combination to satisfying sex may be the foods you eat—and herbs too.

Research suggests that some neurotransmitters, including dopamine, norepinephrine, and acetylcholine, may stimulate and sustain one's sex drive. These neurotransmitters work in tandem with ample amounts of vitamins C, E, and the B's, and the mineral zinc.

Along with a good supply of these nutrients and neurotransmitters, a low intake of fat and cholesterol makes a big difference, especially for men. As you already know, too much fat and cholesterol can clog blood vessels and reduce blood flow. Just as a blocked artery to the heart can bring on a heart attack, blocked vessels to the genitals can interfere with sexual function.

Statistics indicate that impotence increases in midlife, and by age sixty, one out of every four men no longer has sex. Eating meat increases the likelihood of impotency, primarily because it's full of cholesterol and saturated fats.

High blood pressure seems to interfere with satisfying sex too. A study of 211 premenopausal women, half of whom had hypertension, showed that the women with high blood pressure experienced less vaginal lubrication and more difficulty achieving orgasm.

Whatever your gender, taking medicinal herbs may fire up your libido. Ginseng, for instance, has been used in Asia as a sexual tonic for thousands of years. It's believed to boost libido in general and to increase vaginal lubrication. Ginkgo biloba improves blood flow.

If sexual difficulties persist, consult a doctor or other health practitioner.

almost vegetarians who power-eat can most definitely live long.

And live very well.

■ NO MORE CANCER OR OSTEOPOROSIS ■

Or heart disease, stroke, adult-onset diabetes, obesity, or other chronic illnesses.

Does this sound too good to be true?

Well, maybe it is. We all know people who took good care of themselves, ate right (lots of grains, vegetables, fruits, and legumes), exercised regularly, and made smart lifestyle choices like maintaining friendships and staying away from cigarettes. Yet they endured a chronic illness or died early in life.

I think of my friend Audrey. In her late thirties, she noticed that swallowing felt strangely uncomfortable, and she made a doctor's appointment, suspecting a minor infection or some other no-biggie health problem.

But chest X-rays told a different story: lung cancer.

DO YOU NEED A SUPPLEMENT?

If you measured the health of Americans based on the number of bottles of vitamins and minerals lining pharmacy shelves, you'd come to this conclusion: We're the best nourished—or the most health-nutty—people on the planet.

The truth is, most Americans do not even get the recommended five to nine servings of vegetables and fruits a day. Only 20 percent eat the minimal five. And so some of us swallow more than ten billion tablets—round ones, oval-shaped ones, capsules, miniature Pebbles and BamBams—at a cost of $700 million each year.

But are supplements truly necessary? Do you need one?

The purists say food can provide you with all the vitamins and minerals you need to power your mind, mood, and body. Certainly a sound diet makes nutritional sense.

Let's say you are eating right: Your foods are varied, you get sufficient calories, and your meals are vegetarian or nearly so. Yet you want a boost. Maybe you feel blue, are fatigued, or just don't feel quite up to par.

New scientific research is showing that supplements can help good eaters too.

By now, you've heard that taking in adequate folic acid, a B vitamin, helps prevent neurological birth defects like spina bifida. What you may not know is that tiny deficiencies of some nutrients can contribute to depression, tiredness, premenstrual migraines, poor memory, fuzzy thinking, and other symptoms.

With so many supplements from which to choose, it's difficult to know what to do. Keep this in mind: It's dangerous to overdose. Though death from overdose is rare, some gung-ho pill poppers suffer side effects, ranging from nausea and dizziness to tooth loss and liver damage.

So how much is safe?

Jeffrey Blumberg, Ph.D., professor of nutrition at Tufts University, gives these guidelines:

It's fine to take 10 to 20 milligrams of beta-carotene, 250 to 1,000 milligrams of vitamin C, and 100 to 400 IU of vitamin E each day. With the exception of vitamins A and D (for which you should not exceed the Recommended Dietary Allowances [RDAs]), taking up to double the RDAs of the other vitamins and minerals is considered safe.

Like all medication, keep supplements out of the reach of children. (Just one or two iron tablets can kill a little one.) And if you have any questions or concerns, consult your doctor or health practitioner.

It made no sense. She had never smoked or lived with smokers. She'd never held a job that put her at risk for lung cancer. Rather, she ate well and was active. She was exceptionally close to her husband, children, parents, and friends.

To eke out as many years as possible, she followed doctor's orders, receiving radiation treatments and chemotherapy. For a short while, it appeared she was out of the woods—her cancer was in remission. Then it spread rapidly to her bones and brain. She died shortly after her fortieth birthday.

Why Audrey? Why does anyone who has taken good care of herself die of a horrible illness?

I don't pretend to have the answer. All I know is life's not fair. The good die young sometimes, while the bad often live long and well—or so it seems. I could offer a sermon on why we get sick and die, but I'll save it for another book.

My point is that power-eating gives you a tremendous edge in living long and living well. So do regular exercise and close ties to family and friends. But they're no guarantees. When your number's up, that's it.

Before this gets morbid, let's rewind to the "tremendous edge" part.

Study after study confirm that vegetarians and almost vegetarians not only outlive meat-eating folks by several years on average, but also suffer fewer chronic and other illnesses.

How come? What's the secret behind power-eating, exercise, and close relationships?

In two words, strong immunity.

■ Building Immunity ■

Think of your immune system as a squadron of guardian angels, ready to defend and protect you from "evils"—like cancer, heart disease, infection, even the common cold—whether they attack from outside your body or from within. With a strong immune system, you are less likely to become ill, and if you happen to land in the sickbed, you're back on your feet relatively quickly.

But when the wear and tear of daily living weakens your immune system—an unfortunate (but not guaranteed!) result of aging—your body becomes an easy target.

A relatively new field of nutritional immunology is investigating how food and its components support the unbelievably complicated immune system. Though tabloids shout "7 Foods for Perfect Immunity" and newscasters trumpet so-called miraculous findings that red wine, garlic, and tofu could keep you healthy forever and a day, researchers see the truth: The immune system still remains a mystery.

WALK AWAY FROM ILLNESS

When you have a cold, is it smart to exercise?

The folks in the white coats are saying yes. Research studies since the late 1980s show that activity and exercise at moderate levels build immunity. In one study, researchers at Appalachian State University in North Carolina tested women in their thirties and found that those who walked briskly for forty-five minutes, five days a week, for four months during peak cold season got fewer colds than women who didn't exercise. The walkers were sick with colds for only five days on average during the four months, while their sedentary peers reported double that amount. (By the way, breathing cold air kills many of the viruses that live in the nose.)

Excited by these findings, the same researchers conducted a similar experiment with women in their sixties, seventies, and eighties. Half of them walked thirty-seven minutes a day, five days a week, over three months; the others didn't exercise. The results: 50 percent of the nonexercisers caught colds; only 21 percent of the walkers did.

How does exercise rev up the immune system?

Scientists say that within minutes of a physical activity—be it walking, polishing the floor by hand, or cleaning out gutters—an exerciser's white blood cells increase in number. White blood cells are an essential part of the squadron of "guardian angels" that defend your body against invaders like bacteria and viruses.

Your white blood cell count returns to preexercise levels within a few hours. But the temporary boost has day-long benefits, helping the immune system to run more efficiently. When you walk, cycle, or swim, the body releases two hormones—adrenaline and cortisol—which trigger your health-promoting T-cell lymphocytes.

What's becoming clear is that aerobic exercise—the kind that works the cardiovascular system—is the best for charging up the immune system's ability to fight disease.

But hang in there.

An avalanche of studies are unearthing some clues, delicious clues, showing the unmistakable value of power-eating, activity, exercise, (covered extensively in chapter 8) and close ties to family and friends.

Here's a quickie quiz to gauge how much you already know about building strong immunity:

1. The most powerful antioxidants are beta-carotene, selenium, and vitamins C and B_{12}. *True False*
2. All free radicals are bad. *True False*
3. Alzheimer's victims are short on the neurotransmitter acetylcholine. *True False*
4. When you have a cold or a sore back, or are recovering from cancer, you should get lots of rest and minimal activity to strengthen your immunity. *True False*
5. Married couples as a whole live longer and remain healthier than single people. *True False*

The answers: *1. False.* B_{12} is not considered an antioxidant. *2. False.* Free radicals generate energy you need to live. *3. True.* Acetylcholine is the memory-managing neurotransmitter. *4. False.* Activity stimulates your immune system. *5. True.* On average married couples live significantly longer than single people.

FREE RADICALS REVISITED

To protect your memory and age-proof your brain, think antioxidants. This buzzword of the early nineties got lots of people talking about vitamins C and E, beta-carotene, and selenium and swiping bottles of them from pharmacy shelves.

Antioxidants neutralize oxidants. Oxidants (hereafter referred to as free radicals) are the Darth Vaders in the story of aging. Free radicals mess with your neurons and other body cells. They make your skin sag, your bones creak, and your mind falter.

Because free radicals carry an unpaired electron, they are unstable and steal electrons from other molecules, creating more free radicals. If antioxidants fail to stop the biochemical kleptomaniacs, the dangerous chain reaction continues unabated. Any molecule can be a target. This includes the fats in cell membranes, mitochondria (the power center of cells), and DNA.

Here's my favorite word picture of the effect of free radicals on aging: A mass of glowing lightbulbs, representing active neurons, fills a room. Then a golf ball is tossed into it, bouncing here and there and knocking out a few lights. At first, the room is still bright because many lights are still shining. But as the golf ball continues its wild travels, more lights break and the room dims.

CHECKERS, ANYONE?

One of the best ways to stay mentally sharp as the years go by is to play games. Crossword puzzles, poker, Pictionary, chess, mancala, Scrabble, checkers—any game that makes you think scores high in keeping you young.

Research indicates that regular game players build more complex webs of neural connections in the brain than do those who think games are for kids only. What's more, the more neural connections you have, the more mentally agile you're likely to be later in life.

That's right: Playing games is as valuable to a strong mind as exercise is to a strong body.

In a landmark study that led to programs such as Head Start and educational television shows including *Sesame Street*, rats that were given toys and played together learned to navigate mazes far quicker than did rats who lived in unfun cages. The rats showed differences in their cerebral cortex: This part of the brain largely concerned with thought was significantly thicker in the toy-happy rats.

Researchers say this finding applies not only to rats and children but to adults as well. Mental stimulation boosts brain power at any age. It's no surprise then that research strongly suggests that people who have attended college and/or have held mentally challenging jobs are less likely to develop dementia.

Incidentally, watching games seems to have no positive effect on brain power. You've got to play. So next time you're tempted to view reruns of the sitcom *Friends*, find a friend and challenge him to a game of, well, you figure it out.

But free radicals aren't all bad.

The body uses them to produce energy for all of our activities, from sleeping to working. Ironically, the major source of free radical production is breathing.

The way free radicals cause aging is at least threefold:

First, free radicals attach to fats in cell membranes, damaging their structure and function. The cells can no longer absorb nutrients, oxygen, and water, and after repeated attacks, the cells are made useless. The cell membranes rupture and leak the cells' contents, damaging the surrounding tissues.

Second, free radicals mess with mitochondria if they can get to them, causing the cells to stop producing energy and, finally, to die. Only cell remnants remain, accumulating around neurons and interfering with their message-sending jobs.

Third, free radicals hook onto DNA, which regulates cell reproduction, risking the body's genetic code. The damage may kill the cell or alter it so that its genetic code cannot be read. Free radicals also attack RNA, which receives instructions from the DNA.

But wait. Here comes Luke Skywalker to battle Darth Vader. Antioxidants neutralize free radicals, making them as harmless as dandelion fluff. By neutralizing free radicals, antioxidant nutrients can control the rate of damage to body cells and, in turn, slow aging and ultimately senility.

For instance, Ranjit Chandra, the pioneering scientist in nutritional immunology at the Memorial University in Newfoundland, has probed the link between what we eat and how we age and has documented that the more antioxidants you take in, the stronger your immunity.

In a study of eighty-six healthy, independently living men and women, Chandra found that those who were given multivitamin-and-mineral supplements that contained doses of antioxidants slightly higher than the Recommended Daily Allowances fared better than those who were given a placebo (a look-alike capsule with no nutrients). The supplement-takers were sick with infection-related illness a little less than half as much as the placebo-takers. The supplement-takers also showed significant improvement in seven measures of immune function, including their ability to produce antibodies in response to a flu vaccine.

The main nutrient antioxidants are beta-carotene and vitamins C and E. Beta-carotene, found in sweet potatoes, carrots, peaches, spinach, and other yellow-orange and dark green vegetables and fruits, is turned into vitamin A in the small intestine and prevents the formation of many highly reactive free radicals. Most prevalent in citrus, vitamin C stands guard in and around cells to prevent damage by free radicals. Vitamin E, found in nuts, oils, and wheat germ, protects cell membranes by scavenging free radicals before they attack the fat in cell membranes. This is critical to the brain, which is about 60 percent fat.

Joining these nutrient antioxidants is selenium, a mineral necessary to the formation of an enzyme that fights free radicals. You can find selenium in such foods as grains, egg yolks, milk, cheese, fresh garlic, wheat germ, broccoli, cabbage, mushrooms, onion, and Brazil nuts (its richest source—just one or two Brazil nuts meets the Recommended Dietary Allowance for this mineral).

That's just part of the good-guy team. Other antioxidants include flavonoids (such as tannins in tea, garlic, and the herb ginseng). Expect to hear more about newly discovered antioxidants in the years to come. This area of research is red-hot.

What's the ideal intake of antioxidants?

Studies have used varying amounts, from the Recommended Dietary Allowance (RDA) to megadoses. Looking at the data, the editorial board of the *UC Berkeley Wellness Letter* updated its position on supplements, recommending that adults consume 6 to 15 milligrams (mg) of beta-carotene daily, 250 to 500mg of vitamin C, and 200 to 800 International Units (IU) of vitamin E.

Though these amounts appear harmless, consult your doctor or health practitioner before supplementing your diet. Always steer clear of megadoses of other vitamins and minerals. They can be toxic in high doses.

Of course, pills cannot replace good foods.

So start with the Power-Up Food Plan in chapter 7 and consider supplementation, if indicated, for extra protection against an aging brain with fewer neurons to store, access, and transfer information, and, believe it or not, old-looking skin.

Research suggests that eating an antioxidant-rich diet and taking supplements, specifically vitamin E, may protect against photoaging. Though antioxidants won't make a fifty-year-old's skin look like a twenty-year-old's, they can help you look more youthful and lower your risk of skin cancer.

FIVE ANTIAGING GUIDELINES

To boost your immunity through food:

1. Eat extra fruits and vegetables. These treasures supply a wealth of antioxidants and phytochemicals. The government's recommendation stands at five to nine servings a day. Get at least this much if not more.

2. Pile on the beans. Research shows that people

THE ANTIAGING SCOREBOARD

To think, act, and feel years younger than the age on your driver's license, eat antioxidants. The four best recognized antioxidants are beta-carotene, vitamins C and E, and the mineral selenium. They help neutralize free radicals, which contribute to disease and other signs of aging, including wrinkles.

Below are many foods with antioxidant power. Be sure to get no less than the Recommended Dietary Allowance (RDA).

VITAMIN A
The RDA for vitamin A, the precursor to beta-carotene, is 800 RE (retinol equivalents) for women and 1,000 mcg RE for men.

Pumpkin (½ cup mashed, boiled): 2,691 mcgRE
Sweet potato (1 medium, baked): 2,488 mcgRE
Carrot (1 medium, raw): 2,025 mcgRE
Mango (1 medium): 806 mcgRE
Spinach (½ cup, boiled): 737 mcgRE
Butternut squash (½ cup cubes, boiled): 714 mcgRE
Papaya (1 medium): 612 mcgRE
Cantaloupe (1 cup pieces): 516 mcgRE
Kale (½ cup chopped, boiled): 481 mcgRE
Peach (10 halves, dried): 281 mcgRE
Apricot (10 halves, dried): 253 mcgRE
Tomato (1 medium, raw): 139 mcgRE

VITAMIN C
The RDA is 60mg (milligrams) for men and women, although many nutritionists think it should be much higher.

Red bell pepper (½ cup chopped, raw): 95mg
Strawberries (1 cup): 85mg
Orange (1 medium): 80mg
Kiwi (1 medium) 75mg

Green bell peppers (½ cup chopped, raw): 64mg

Brussels sprouts (4 sprouts, boiled): 46mg

Grapefruit (½ medium): 47mg

Broccoli (½ cup chopped, raw): 41mg

Cauliflower (½ cup pieces, raw): 36mg

Lotus root (10 slices, raw): 36mg

Sweet potato (1 medium, baked): 28mg

Kale (½ cup, boiled): 27mg

Potato (1 medium, baked, with skin): 26mg

Collards (½ cup, boiled): 23mg

Tomato (1 medium, raw): 22mg

Red cabbage (½ cup, shredded, raw): 20mg

Asparagus (6 spears, boiled): 18mg

VITAMIN E

The RDA is 8 mg (milligrams) for women and 10mg for men.

Hazelnuts (1 ounce): 6.7mg

Almonds (1 ounce): 6.5mg

Wheat germ (¼ cup): 6mg

Safflower oil (1 tablespoon): 4.6mg

Peanut butter (1 tablespoon): 3mg

Whole-wheat flour (⅓ cup): 3mg

Corn oil (1 tablespoon): 2mg

SELENIUM

The RDA is 55mcg (micrograms) for women and 70mcg for men.

Brazil nuts (1 nut): 50mcg

Brown rice (½ cup, cooked): 13mcg

Egg (1 large): 12mcg

Whole-wheat bread (1 slice): 11mcg

Milk (1 cup): 3.6mcg

Peanuts (¼ cup): 3mcg

Wheat germ (¼ cup): 10mcg

Broccoli (½ cup, cooked): 7mcg

Cabbage (½ cup, raw): 6.5mcg

Mushrooms (½ cup, raw): 7mcg

Onion (¼ cup, cooked): 5mcg

who include legumes of all sorts—and especially soybeans—in their daily fare tend to live longer and have fewer illnesses than those who don't.

3. Savor ample (not excessive) amounts of mineral-rich foods. When minerals like copper, iron, selenium, and zinc are in short supply, your immune system weakens. The same may be true when you get too much by taking high-dose supplements. More is not always better. Think balance.

4. Shelve the sugar. Studies have documented the suppression of the immune system in the hours after eating sweets or sugar-laced foods or drinks. If you have chocolate or ice cream on occasion, eat it at one sitting, not throughout the day, to allow your immune system to rebound.

5. Go easy on fat. Eating more fat than 20 to 25 percent of total calories appears to suppress the immune system. Some researchers say that includes the "good" fats (monounsaturated and polyunsaturated) too.

When you practice these immunity-boosting guidelines (in other words, when you power-eat, as outlined in my Power-Up Food Plan), you'll probably get ample age-proofing nutrients.

I say "probably" because many older people, as well as young or middle-aged adults, have mild to moderate vitamin and mineral deficiencies. Usually they do not know it. And yet the deficiency of one or more nutrients can have a profound effect on body power—and brain and mood power too.

An example is vitamin D. Termed "the silent epidemic" by the Center for Science in the Public Interest, a Washington, D.C.–based consumer advocacy group, vitamin D deficiency is a leading contributor to osteoporosis, which affects some 25 million Americans.

Vitamin D's main function is to maintain a healthy level of blood calcium. It does that by telling the intestines to absorb more calcium from the food you eat. If you're vitamin D deficient, your body can't get enough calcium for its needs even when your diet has an ample amount of this mineral. The result is accelerated bone loss and increased risk for fractures that debilitate and may lead to death.

And don't forget: Vitamins and minerals work hand in hand with your neurotransmitters, which pass on important messages among your neurons, or brain cells. Research shows that even a mild deficiency in a nutrient puts a damper on the function of neurotransmitters, possibly causing impaired thinking, poor mood, and compromised physical performance.

That goes for one of the most obvious signs of aging: poor memory.

NOW WHERE DID I PUT THE CAR KEYS?

Almost everyone knows someone whose memory is fading like autumn leaves in November. One of my friends watched her accomplished mother transform into a confused, aged woman who would set the table for five when no company was expected. Another friend, too, noticed that his nonagenarian mother could no longer remember the time or the day or the month or the year. She worried excessively. Still another witnessed the deterioration of a woman he visited weekly at a nursing home. At first she had little difficulty remembering things, whether important or unimportant. Within a year, she couldn't even recall his name.

No doubt you're aware of Ronald Reagan's bout with Alzheimer's disease and his wife's campaign to get the word out about this degenerative disorder. Its symptoms are gradual loss of memory of recent events and the inability to learn new information; a growing tendency to repeat oneself, misplace objects, and get lost; a loss in good judgment and social graces; and an increase in irritability, anxiety, and depression.

Until recently, a vitamin B–like compound called choline was not seen as essential to health. New evidence suggests the opposite. Choline might be a premier ingredient for brain development and function—and it may be at the root of age-related memory loss.

Choline is a building block for the memory-managing neurotransmitter acetylcholine. Average daily intake is 700 to 1,000 milligrams; deficiency symptoms—memory loss and unclear thinking, for instance—arise when intake falls below this amount. If you don't take in enough choline from food—no matter what your age—your brain power suffers. Your brain cannot store or retrieve information, and you experience minor aggravation to complete debilitation.

Your brain can make some of its own choline with the help of vitamin B_{12} and folic acid, but it needs a boost from food for optimal functioning. Choline-rich foods include eggs, wheat germ, and soybeans.

It's never too soon to chow down choline-rich foods. In one study, older patients showed improvement in long-term memory when they took in 35 grams of lecithin daily for four to six weeks. Scientists caution that choline supplementation is probably most useful in the early stages of memory loss, before structural changes in the brain cause irreversible damage.

When you eat too little choline, your memory as well as your overall thinking is at risk. In one study, people given a drug that blocked acetylcholine function flunked memory tests, while those given an acetylcholine-boosting drug passed easily.

And while you're upping your choline intake, keep away from meats. Though more research is needed, it appears that homocysteine, an amino acid found at high levels in the bloodstream of people who eat meat regularly, is linked to a type of mental disorientation often seen in the early stages of Alzheimer's disease.

The take-to-the-kitchen message: Eat healthy vegetarian meals that include choline-rich foods (even the lowly egg!) for better memory now and when you're collecting Social Security.

FRIEND TO FRIEND

How long and well you live may have their beginnings in your diaper days. Research indicates that the more loving and affectionate your early childhood, the better. But even if you didn't grow up in a loving home, you can increase your chances for greater longevity and well-being in the decades to come by making this choice: Don't be a loner.

The diaper-days theory suggests that frequent hugs between mother (or dad or auntie) and child may be a factor in how long and well you live, and a little extra stimulation may matter significantly to brain development. In one study, researchers tracked men into their sixties to find out what early factors, such as scholastic achievement and regular exercise, would predict the men's physical and mental well-being at retirement.

Surprisingly, topping the list was a "warm childhood environment" and not whether one had smoked, exercised regularly, or had octogenarian ancestors.

Along the same lines, research shows that children who received extra attention from their parents or other permanent caregivers outperform their playmates who lack close family ties. The latter also have a poorer self-image that often follows them into adulthood. The probable result: Negativity and stress toys with the immune system, paving the way for health problems later in life.

In addition, loving touches and an opportunity to safely explore one's surroundings might help the brain to put a brake on certain types of stress responses. For instance, gamma aminobutyric acid (or GABA) functions in the brain as an inhibitory neurotransmitter. In other words, it tones down brain activity. Having too little GABA or too many GABA receptors may contribute to anxiety. Some researchers speculate that cumulative stress starting in a strict, unloving home may create disturbances in GABA function. Conversely, both the endorphins and serotonin increase when a person is given affirmation.

No matter your genetics and childhood experiences, you can enhance your chances for longevity and well-being by surrounding yourself with friends and family. Social scientists have known for decades that isolated people tend to die at an earlier age than those with fuller social calendars. A leading researcher has reviewed key data and concluded "a lack of social relationships constitutes a major risk factor for mortality."

In a landmark study, researchers surveyed 4,776 people in Alameda County in California about their marriage status, contacts with friends and family, church membership, and other group affiliations. They found that the low scorers on the combined "social network index" were twice as likely to die in the next nine years. Another study found similar results: The death rate was two to three times higher for unsociable men and about two times higher for unsociable women among two thousand adults surveyed in Tecumseh, Michigan.

If ever you needed a reason to rekindle a friendship or join the PTA, you've got one now. The adage that there's safety in numbers certainly holds true for living longer and living better.

And teach it to your children. The more loving their home, the happier and healthier they will be for many, many years to come. When you model to them the value of exercising and having friends, they're even better off. And showing them how to power-eat deliciously takes the cake for sure—Raspberry Cheese Crumb Cake, that is. The recipe is on page 303.

Enjoy.

■ THE LIVE-LONG CUSTOMIZER ■

1. Eat live-long foods. Here are examples:

LIVE-LONG FOODS	LIVE-LESS-LONG FOODS
Beta-carotene biggies, such as yellow-orange produce like cantaloupe and sweet potatoes	Junk food
	Lots of sugar
	Meat daily
High-C sweeties like oranges, strawberries, and green leafies	Fat intake at 30 percent or more of daily calories
Vitamin E wonders, such as whole grains, oils, nuts, and seeds in moderation	
Selenium supers, such as whole grains and vegetables	
Phytochemicals, found abundantly in vegetables and fruits	

As you'll recall, certain life choices figure in to longevity, including having strong friendships, being active, and reducing stress when possible.

2. Eat live-long foods at the right times.
Any time is the right time for live-long foods. So try to eat them at every meal and snack.

3. Eat live-long foods in the right combos.
Any combo works well.

Live-long tip of the day: Power-eat day in and day out until it becomes so natural that it's life.

## II

How to Power Up

If I had but two loaves of bread,
I would sell one
and buy hyacinths, for they
would feed my soul.

—THE KORAN

The Power-Up Food Plan

Have you ever baked a loaf of bread? I don't mean the ready-to-pop-in-the-oven pretenders in your grocer's refrigerators and freezers. I mean from scratch.

You know, flour up to your elbows, a bit of salt and sweetener, warm water, and . . . and . . .

The yeast.

Never forget the yeast! Without this ingredient, all of your measuring, mixing, kneading, shaping, rising, and proofing is a waste of time. Unless you have a taste for bricks. Nutritious bricks, but bricks just the same.

Like yeast, this chapter and the ones to come give a "lift," a shape, a design to the previous pages of *Energy Eating*. If you're just hopping into these pages, welcome. But I've got a challenge for you. As you read the upcoming pages, spend some time also in part 1 of this book. The first six chapters give a sense of structure to the design of my Power-Up Food Plan, which I'll detail in a moment.

I compare part 1 to gluten—the substance in bread that makes a stretchy structure so your yeasted masterpiece can rise high. Without gluten, you've got glob.

You need the gluten and the yeast, the shape and the substance. With both of them, you get a lifelong membership in the power-eaters' club.

▪ THE PROMISE REVISITED ▪

Energy Eating—the why, the how, and the one-hundred-plus recipes—is the first book to pull together pioneering research findings that are pointing to the once-unthinkable: To boost your brain, lift your mood, and achieve peak physical performance, eat.

More specifically, power-eat.

As mentioned, power-eating is choosing foods to cause a desired effect via your neurotransmitters, those biochemical messengers that pass important chunks of information among your neurons, or brain cells. Every day researchers are fine-tuning their knowledge of how food affects your mind, mood, and body. Here's a taste.

Want to sidestep the postlunch slump? Eat a bowl of protein-rich three-bean chili at noon. Feeling uptight? Enjoy a blueberry muffin and juice. Low on energy? Go for a veggie burger with all the fixin's.

The pioneering research into neurotransmitters and food heralds the power-eating promise: Eating the right foods at the right times in the right combinations powers up your mind, mood, and body—with delicious results.

▪ BRAIN POWER ▪

- clearer, quicker thinking
- greater concentration
- more mental energy
- better memory
- overall mental acuity

▪ MOOD POWER ▪

- stable emotions
- more positive feelings
- an ease in PMS

- less anxiety
- less depression
- overall mood boost

■ BODY POWER ■

- reduced risk for colds and flus as well as heart disease, cancer, and many other chronic diseases
- more physical energy
- greater strength
- faster reaction time
- stronger immunity
- overall physical excellence

It's about time to put the power-eating promise into practice.

■ THE ANATOMY OF THE PLAN ■

Before taking a sneak peek at the Ultimate, the premier version of my Power-Up Food Plan, let me tell you about the Power-Up Food Plan's other big benefits:

- two transition versions—"Getting Started" and "Almost There." They show you how to move successfully from your current eating style to the delicious Ultimate.
- the Power-Up Food Journal—in which you track your meals and snacks for at least three days. This will pinpoint your good and not-so-good eating patterns.
- the Power-Up Food Plan Pyramid—a visual depiction of the Power-Up Food Plan. Photocopy it and hang it on your fridge, at work, anywhere you need a reminder of exceptional eating.
- the Power-Up food families—complete with charts. You'll hear why these families make scientific and gastronomic

sense. The charts of foods and serving sizes are especially helpful in choosing just the right foods for you.

Now for the sneak peek.

■ THE ULTIMATE ■

Every day, eat:

8 to 12 servings of **grains** (with at least half from whole sources).
3 to 6 servings of **vegetables** (including one high in beta-carotene and one "super veggie").
2 to 5 servings of **fruits** (including one high in vitamin C).
1 to 3 servings of **legumes.**
½ to 2 servings of **nuts and seeds.**
0 to 2 servings of **dairy foods.** (If you have none, take in calcium from other sources. See "Calcium Minus the Cow," page 174.)
0 to 1 serving of **eggs and meat.**
A modest amount of **fats and sweets,** with a maximum of 20 to 25 percent of total calories from fat and no more than 10 percent of total calories from refined sugars. (For a person eating 2,000 calories a day, this means 44 to 56 grams of fat and a max of 50 grams of refined sugar.)
Extras from the grain, vegetable, and fruit families to fill out your calorie needs.
6 to 8 glasses of **water** or the equivalent. (See "Drink Up," page 109.)
A favorite treat of moderate proportions if desired. (Example: one scoop of ice cream, not three scoops smothered in hot fudge!)
I will explain the terms used here in greater detail later.

Did you notice the names of the food families as you perused the Ultimate? Grains, vegetables, fruits, legumes . . . even eggs and meat? These are a far cry from the U.S. Department of Agriculture's (USDA) now infamous basic four food groups of breads and cereals, milk, meat, and vegetables and fruits. The basic four food groups, with half of them pushing animal foods, was science's answer to the deficiency diseases of old.

Enamored with the newly discovered vitamins of the 1900s and vexed by ailments like pellagra (caused by too little niacin in the diet), the nutritionists' knee-jerk response was to tell people to eat like kings. The meat and dairy lobbies put in more than their two cents' worth, and the basic four food groups were born.

Then came the new diseases: cancer, heart disease, stroke, osteoporosis, adult-onset (or Type 2) diabetes, and obesity.

These were virtually unheard-of prior to World War II. They are diseases of excess, which follow us like thieves into the twenty-first century, robbing us of our well-being and our lives.

Enough history for now. If you want to learn more, I urge you to read the last third of *The New Laurel's Kitchen,* an excellent vegetarian nutrition and recipe book. It brims with details of the American nutrition triumphs and defeats from the early 1900s through 1985.

As you know, the basic four food groups are out, and the USDA's Food Guide Pyramid is in. But it's got big problems too. (See "The USDA's Problematic Pyramid," page 155.)

Hello, Power-Up Food Plan.

This easy-to-follow plan combines the latest and most reliable scientific knowledge of nutrition with absolutely great taste. And it balances your neurotransmitters: serotonin, dopamine, norepinephrine, the endorphins, acetylcholine, and others. Remember: Your neurotransmitters can make or break how well you think, feel, and perform. Without them, you couldn't even lift a finger, literally.

For the sake of your neurotransmitters, the power-eating promise centers on *what* you eat and *how* you eat (the timing of your meals and the combinations of foods in your meals). There's no better way to key in to your personal eating style than by a simple and accurate method of journaling.

THE POWER-UP FOOD PLAN PYRAMID

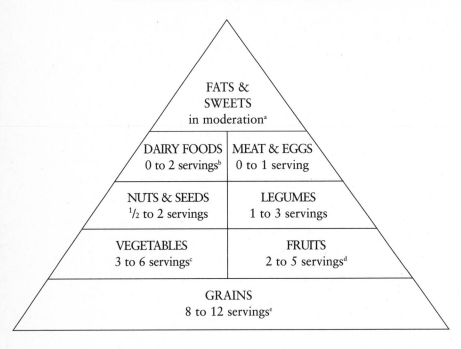

FATS &
SWEETS
in moderation[a]

DAIRY FOODS | MEAT & EGGS
0 to 2 servings[b] | 0 to 1 serving

NUTS & SEEDS | LEGUMES
$\frac{1}{2}$ to 2 servings | 1 to 3 servings

VEGETABLES | FRUITS
3 to 6 servings[c] | 2 to 5 servings[d]

GRAINS
8 to 12 servings[e]

[a]**Fats & Sweets:** Your fat calories should range from 20 to 25 percent of your total calories, or about 44 to 56 grams, for a person eating 2,000 total calories a day. Calories from refined sugars should not exceed 10 percent of your total calories, or about 50 grams (which is equal to about 12 teaspoons) for a person eating 2,000 total calories daily.

[b]**Dairy Foods:** If you eat none, be sure to eat high-calcium plant foods. (See "Calcium Minus the Cow," page 174.)

[c]**Vegetables:** Choose one high in beta-carotene (e.g., sweet potatoes, carrots, and dark leafy greens). Also choose one "super" vegetable.

[d]**Fruits:** Choose one high in vitamin C (e.g., citrus fruits, kiwifruit, and watermelon).

[e]**Grains:** At least half of your selections should be whole, not refined. Examples include bran cereal, whole-grain breadstuffs, oatmeal, and brown rice.

▪ THE POWER-UP FOOD JOURNAL ▪

The power-up food journal (see page 158) is as essential to a new power-eater as a night out *alone* is to the parents of toddlers.

Basically, it's a record of what and how you eat, and your moods too, right now, *before* you begin the delightful adventure of power-eating. You unveil your current eating style—the strengths and the weaknesses—so you know where you are and where you need to go.

For example, let's say your power-up food journal shows that you already eat lots of vegetables and fruits, including the ones high in vitamin C and beta-carotene (congrats!), but your grain selections are "refined" and rarely "whole," and you eat twice as much fat and refined sugar than is ideal. Because you have several areas to improve, go straight to the Getting Started version and ease into power-eating gracefully.

THE USDA'S PROBLEMATIC PYRAMID

Is the USDA's Food Guide Pyramid better than the infamous four food groups? Yes, because it puts greater emphasis on eating grains, vegetables, and fruits. Does it show you the best way to eat? Not a chance.

The main problem with the USDA's Food Guide Pyramid is that it fails to address America's problem of excess. For instance, according to the Food Guide Pyramid you could eat a nine-ounce slab of steak each day and feel righteous, because it allows three three-ounce servings of meat daily. The meat alone is about 60 grams of fat, much of it saturated, 250 milligrams of cholesterol, and nearly 900 calories.

Worse, the Food Guide Pyramid makes no distinction between refined versus whole grains or between marginally nutritious versus exceptional vegetables and fruits. In terms of the Pyramid, Wonder bread is on par with whole-grain loaves and iceberg lettuce equals the dark leafy greens. Any nutritionist worth her salt would disagree.

The truth is, the Food Guide Pyramid might as well tumble down or undergo major reconstruction. That's not only my opinion but also that of the Center for Science in the Public Interest—a Washington, D.C.–based consumer advocacy group—and other nutritionally aware scientists and groups, including Oldways Preservation & Exchange Trust, which has developed four of its own food pyramids: Mediterranean, Asian, Latin American, and "healthy, traditional vegetarian diet."

One scientist even charged that the Food Guide Pyramid might cause more heart attacks.

Or suppose you eat lots of vegetables and fruits, and at least half of your grain selections are "whole." You're even eating a health-smart amount of minimal refined sugars, but you overdose on dairy products and have a love affair with butter. With a few areas to improve, you may skip Getting Started and jump to the Almost There version because, well, you're almost there.

Or if you adore whole grains, vegetables, and fruits, you go easy on fats and refined sugars, and you eat healthy amounts of dairy products, eggs, and nuts and seeds. But you rarely eat protein- and nutrient-rich legumes. The Ultimate is where you may begin, because your eating style needs only fine-tuning.

So how do you keep a power-up food journal?

First, make three to five photocopies of "My Power-Up Food Journal" or jot it down on separate sheets of paper.

Second, for three to five days, write down *everything* you eat and drink, even the jelly beans from your co-worker's candy dish, and record the time, food amount, moods, and thoughts before the meal or snack and thirty minutes after, and your state of hunger before eating.

Third, tally the type and amount of food you ate in each of the following categories: grains, vegetables, fruits, nuts and seeds, legumes, dairy products, eggs and meat, fats, and sweets.

Fourth, look at your lists carefully to answer the following questions. Give yourself a point for each yes answer.

- Did you average at least eight to twelve grain servings daily? Were at least half of your grain serving from whole grains, such as whole wheat, rolled oats, brown rice, bulgur, whole-grain couscous, and wheat berries?
- Did you eat three to six servings of vegetables a day? Was one or more daily serving high in beta-carotene? Was one or more daily serving a "super veggie"? (See "Super Veggies," page 165.)
- Did you eat two to five servings of fruit a day? Was one of your daily servings high in vitamin C?
- Did you eat one to three servings of legumes a day?

- Did you eat one-half to two servings of nuts and/or seeds a day?
- Did you eat zero to two servings of dairy foods a day and if you ate zero did you eat a high-calcium food in its place?
- Did you eat zero to one serving of eggs and/or meat a day?
- Did you eat fats in moderation, keeping fat calories at 20 to 25 percent of total calories? Did you eat refined sugar in moderation, with their calories at no more than 10 percent of total calories?
- Did you drink six to eight glasses of water or the equivalent each day?

Fifth, add up your points. The highest possible score is 14. If you scored 7 or fewer points, begin with the Getting Started version (below) of my Power-Up Food Plan. If you scored 8 to 11 points, choose the Almost There version (page 160). If you scored over 11 points, jump right in to the Ultimate (page 161).

▪ GETTING STARTED ▪

This version eases you in to power-eating at its best. In my wellness counseling, I've observed that the people who improve their food choices step by step are the most likely to succeed and come to experience brain power, mood power, and body power. As they nix excess fat and sugar and make other power-up choices, they enjoy the luxury of trying new foods and learning healthier cooking methods while giving their taste buds time to adjust.

But if you count yourself among the few with a let's-jump-right-in personality style, don't let me hold you back. Go ahead and attempt the Ultimate. But feel free to return to Getting Started—and please don't harbor any guilt if you do return. That's why it's here.

The Getting Started version is quite similar to the Ultimate, but it lets you eat the type and quantities of foods that somewhat approximate your current eating style. I hope you caught my

MY POWER-UP FOOD JOURNAL

date: _____

time	mood & thoughts BEFORE	foods & beverages	amount	hungry?	mood & thoughts AFTER

Grains:
# of total servings _____   # of whole-grain servings _____

Vegetables:
# of total servings _____   # of beta-carotene-rich servings _____
# of super veggie servings _____

Fruits:
# of total servings _____   # of vitamin C–rich servings _____

Nuts and seeds:
# of total servings _____

Legumes:
# of total servings _____

Dairy products:
# of total servings _____
If zero, # of high-calcium, nondairy servings _____

Eggs and meat:
# of total servings _____

Fats and sweets:
# of fat grams _____   # of refined sugar grams _____

qualifier. Though it *somewhat* approximates how you eat today, it still pushes you up, as in power-*up*.

Every day, eat:

6 to 12 servings of **grains** (with at least two servings from whole sources).

3 to 6 servings of **vegetables** (including one high in beta-carotene).

2 to 5 servings of **fruits** (including one high in vitamin C).

½ to 1 serving of **legumes.**

0 to 2 servings of **nuts and seeds.**

0 to 3 servings of **dairy foods.** (If you have none, take in calcium from other sources. See "Calcium Minus the Cow," page 174.)

0 to 2 servings of **eggs and meat.**

A modest amount of **fats and sweets,** with a maximum of 30 percent of total calories from fat and no more than 20 percent of total calories from refined sugars. (For a person eating 2,000 calories a day, this means a max of 67 grams of fat and 100 grams of refined sugar.)

Extras from the grain, vegetable, and fruit families to fill out your calorie needs.

At least 4 glasses of **water** or the equivalent.

1 to 2 favorite treats of moderate proportions if desired.

Follow the Getting Started version until you're comfortable with it. One way you can gauge your comfort is by filling out a few more blank copies of "My Power-Up Food Journal" and see whether you're right on target with the Getting Started goals without feeling deprived. This may take a week or a couple of months, depending on your eating habits before power-eating, your personality style, and a host of other factors.

Then move on to Almost There.

■ ALMOST THERE ■

This version of my Power-Up Food Plan is a decent eating plan
by almost anyone's standards. It, too, approximates the Ultimate
but it gets you even closer to right where you want to be: cashing
in on the benefits of the power-eating promise.

Every day, eat:

8 to 12 servings of **grains** (with at least three of them from
whole sources).

3 to 6 servings of **vegetables** (including one high in beta-
carotene and one "super veggie").

2 to 5 servings of **fruits** (including one high in vitamin C).

½ to 2 servings of **legumes.**

1 to 2 servings of **nuts and seeds.**

0 to 2 servings of **dairy foods.** (If you have none, take in
calcium from other sources. See "Calcium Minus the
Cow," page 174.)

0 to 1 serving of **eggs and meat.**

A modest amount of **fats and sweets,** with a maximum of 25
percent of total calories from fat and no more than 15 percent of total calories from refined sugars. (For a person
eating 2,000 calories a day, this means a max of 56 grams
of fat and 75 grams of refined sugar.)

Extras from the grain, vegetable, and fruit families to fill out
your calorie needs.

5 to 8 glasses of **water** or the equivalent.

A favorite treat of moderate proportions if desired.

As with Getting Started, follow this version until you feel
comfortable with it and use blank copies of "My Power-Up Food
Journal" to track your progress.

When you're ready, go for the Ultimate.

▪ ACHIEVE THE ULTIMATE ▪

You made it. Congrats! Celebrate your success with a toast as you raise a glass of Not Quite Champagne. (You'll find the recipe on page 289.)

This version of my Power-Up Food Plan is the ideal way to power up every day. The specifics of the Ultimate were outlined earlier in this chapter on page 152.

While you enjoy the Ultimate, hold dear the power-up principles of part 1. Among the most important are eating protein for brain power and carbos only for mood power; avoiding the sugar boogie blues brought on by overdosing on refined sugar; getting enough nutrients overall, especially the B vitamins, iron, and antioxidants; and feeding your body what it needs when you get a biological food craving.

The power-up principles and the Ultimate go hand in hand like soulmates who dance joyfully to the beat of their song, the song of a truly well-fed body and soul.

But that's not all. Invite the families to the party and get to know them well.

▪ WELCOME, FAMILIES ▪

"Eat your broccoli."

"Finish your veggie burger."

"Drink your milk."

The idea of what foods belong on your plate is inextricably bound to personal likes and dislikes, family tradition, and culture. Many Westerners eat cattle. Most Indians don't. Some Koreans consider dog a delicacy. Americans walk them, feed them, and let them sleep at the foot of their beds.

And yet researchers are determining which foods are nutritional diamonds and which pale in comparison—the cubic zirconiums of the bunch. It turns out that the foods eaten regularly by our *great-grandparents* are the ones we ought to eat too.

Whole grains, vegetables, fruits, legumes, nuts and seeds,

some milk, meat occasionally, and a piece of pie once in a while—
this is what our ancestors ate. And yet they took ill, I admit. But
nutrition-related illnesses didn't put them six feet under; more
than likely, viral and bacterial diseases swept through their towns,
showing no mercy on the young or the old, the weak or the
strong.

Now we know about antibiotics and immunizations and san-
itation. So our life expectancies have inched up. Just imagine how
much higher they'd climb if as a group we'd rediscover the goodness of foods like whole grains.

GRAINS, FOR GOODNESS' SAKE

The grains family is at the very foundation of the Power-Up Food
Plan Pyramid (page 154), allowing for the most selections of any
food family, for solid scientific reasons. Staples since ancient
times, grains provide valuable complex carbohydrates. During digestion, the mammoth carbo molecules are broken down to make
glucose molecules. Your brain feeds exclusively on glucose. That
alone is reason enough to load up on grains.

But there's more.

Iron, zinc, magnesium, and many B vitamins make a respectable appearance in whole grains, as does fiber. But not fat (unless
you slather your bread with butter or load your bagel with cream
cheese). Grains on their own contain a slim four calories per
gram, negligible fat, and no cholesterol. (By the way, only animal
foods contain cholesterol, not plant foods.)

Each serving of bread, rice, pasta, and other grains equals one
selection in the Power-Up Food Plan. A serving provides about
75 calories, 15 grams of carbohydrates, 3 grams of protein, less
than 1 gram of fat, no cholesterol, and 2 grams of fiber for whole
grains and about 1 gram of fiber for refined grains. Choose at
least half of your selections from whole grains.

ITEM	SERVING SIZE
Bagel	½ medium
Bread, whole wheat, multigrain, or white	1 slice
Cereal, cold:	
bran flakes	½ cup
Cheerios	1 cup
cornflakes	1 cup
Grape-Nuts	¼ cup
Rice Krispies	1 cup
Wheaties	1 cup
Crackers:	
graham	2 squares
Ritz	6 crackers
saltines	6 crackers
Wheat Thins	8 crackers
Dinner roll	1 small
English muffin	½ muffin
Flour, any type	2½ tablespoons
Oatmeal	½ cup
Pancake	1 medium
Pasta	½ cup, dry
Pita bread	½ pocket
Pretzels:	
rods	2 rods
thin sticks	20 sticks
traditional shape	15 twists

ITEM	SERVING SIZE
Rice	1/3 cup, dry
Tortillas, flour or corn	1 6-inch
Waffle	1 medium
Wheat germ	3 tablespoons

A RAINBOW OF VEGETABLES

All vegetables are carbo- and nutrient-superior to many other foods in the Power-Up Food Plan Pyramid. Yet their nutrition profiles suggest three separate categories: the "super," the low-calorie, and the high-starch.

Eat a variety of selections from these three vegetable categories, selecting a "super" each day. Worry not if you skip your "super" occasionally; just eat an extra portion next time.

"**Super**" vegetables pack in protein (about 5 grams a serving) as well as vitamins (especially beta-carotene and folic acid) and minerals including calcium and iron. They include the dark leafy greens: spinach, kale, collards, beet greens, dandelion greens, mustard greens, turnip greens, and chard.

No doubt you're familiar with spinach, but try the other dark leafies too. Some are slightly bitter; others have a "bite" or are surprisingly mild. A suggestion: Mix together a couple of dark leafies with romaine and iceberg in a salad. Also in the "super" group are broccoli, Brussels sprouts, sea vegetables, bok choy, and okra. These, too, are nutrient-rich.

Low-calorie vegetables give you a lot for your chewing pleasure: taste, crunch, and meganutrients in relation to their calorie contribution to your meals. Among them are cucumbers, celery, green and red bell peppers, zucchini, radishes, jicama, lettuce, and onions. Some of these are teeming with antioxidants and phyto-chemicals.

Root vegetables top the **high-starch** veggie list. Think pota-toes, sweet potatoes, and carrots. Others are the winter squashes:

acorn, butternut, hubbard, pumpkin, and the like. They supply the antioxidants vitamins A and/or C and have respectable amounts of several B vitamins, calcium, magnesium, and iron.

Each serving of vegetables—whether "super," low-calorie, or high-starch—equals one selection in the Power-Up Food Plan. A serving gives you about 20 calories for low-cal, 50 calories for super, and 75 calories for high-starch; 10 grams of carbohydrates; 1 to 5 grams of protein (the dark leafies are the highest); less than 1 gram of fat; no cholesterol; and 1 to 5 grams of fiber. In general, they also are exceptional sources of antioxidants.

> ## SUPER VEGGIES
>
> These nutritional powerhouses pack protein, vitamins, minerals, antioxidants, and phytochemicals. Many are linked to the prevention of disease. Equally important, they're great-tasting. And that's exactly why the recipe section includes so much of them.
>
> Asparagus
> Bok choy
> Broccoli
> Brussels sprouts
> Chard
> Collards
> Greens (beet, dandelion, mustard, turnip)
> Kale
> Okra
> Sea vegetables

(*) indicates a good beta-carotene choice.

(†) indicates a good vitamin C choice.

Note: The serving sizes are for uncooked vegetables. When cooked, dark leafy greens shrink down by about half; other vegetables aren't similarly affected.

ITEM	TYPE	SERVING SIZE
Artichoke	low-calorie	1 medium
Asparagus*	super	6 spears
Bamboo shoots	low-calorie	½ cup
Beans:		
green	low-calorie	½ cup
lima	high-starch	½ cup
Beets	low-calorie	½ cup

ITEM	TYPE	SERVING SIZE
Bok choy*	super	1 cup
Broccoli*	super	½ cup
Brussels sprouts†	super	½ cup
Cabbage:		
green	low-calorie	1 cup
red	low-calorie	1 cup
Carrots*	high-starch	1 medium
Carrot juice*	high-starch	¾ cup
Cauliflower	low-calorie	½ cup
Celery	low-calorie	1 medium
Chard*†	super	1 cup
Collard greens*†	super	1 cup
Corn	high-starch	½ cup
Cucumber	low-calorie	½ cup
Dandelion greens*	super	1 cup
Eggplant	low-calorie	½ cup
Kale*†	super	1 cup
Kohlrabi	low-calorie	½ cup
Leeks	low-calorie	½ cup
Lettuce	low-calorie	1 cup
Mushrooms	low-calorie	½ cup
Mustard greens*†	super	1 cup
Okra†	super	½ cup
Onion	low-calorie	½ cup
Parsnips	high-starch	½ cup
Peas, green	high-starch	½ cup
Peppers:		
sweet, green†	low-calorie	½ cup
sweet, red*†	low-calorie	½ cup
Potato	high-starch	1 medium
Pumpkin*	high-starch	½ cup
Radishes	low-calorie	½ cup
Rhubarb	low-calorie	1 cup
Rutabagas	low-calorie	½ cup
Sea vegetables*†	super	3½ ounces
Spinach*	super	½ cup
Squash:		
summer	low-calorie	½ cup
winter*	high-starch	½ cup

ITEM	TYPE	SERVING SIZE
Sweet potato*	high-starch	1 medium
Tomato†	low-calorie	1 medium
Tomato juice†	low-calorie	¾ cup
Turnip	low-calorie	½ cup
Turnip greens†	super	1 cup
Water chestnuts	low-calorie	½ cup

FRUITS: THE NATURAL DESSERTS

Who needs Oreos when melons are ripe, apples are crisp, and kiwifruit is primed for the eatin'? Fruits are creation's answer to your sweet tooth—almost. I have yet to find a suitable fruity replacement for chocolate.

On the same level of the Power-Up Food Plan Pyramid as vegetables, fruits have lots to offer: vitamins (like beta-carotene, C, and B_6), minerals (especially potassium and magnesium and sometimes iron and calcium), and fiber.

As always, go for variety. With all the fruits available nowadays, you'll have no trouble in making delectable choices.

Each serving of fruit equals one selection in the Power-Up Food Plan. A serving provides about 50 calories, 10 to 15 grams of carbohydrates, less than 1 gram of protein or fat, no cholesterol, and 2 to 3 grams of fiber. In general, fruits also are exceptional sources of antioxidants and phytochemicals.

(*) indicates a good beta-carotene choice.
(†) indicates a good vitamin C choice.
A word about fruit juices: Aim for no more than one serving a day. Because they lack fiber, they're digested quickly, nearly as fast as soda pop.

ITEM	SERVING SIZE
Apple	1 medium
Apple juice	¾ cup

ITEM	SERVING SIZE
Applesauce, unsweetened	¾ cup
Apricots*	
dried	¼ cup
fresh	1 medium
Banana	1 medium
Berries:	
most varieties	½ cup
strawberries†	½ cup
Cantaloupe*†	½ cup
Currants, dried	¼ cup
Dates, dried	¼ cup
Figs, dried	¼ cup
Grapefruit†	½ medium
Grapefruit juice†	¾ cup
Grapes	½ cup
Guava†	1 medium
Honeydew melon†	½ cup
Kiwifruit†	1 medium
Lemon†	1 medium
Lime†	1 medium
Mango*†	1 medium
Nectarine	1 medium
Orange†	1 medium
Orange juice†	¾ cup
Papaya*†	1 medium

ITEM	SERVING SIZE
Peach	1 medium
Pear	1 medium
Persimmon†	1 medium
Pineapple†	½ cup
Plantain†	1 medium
Plum	1 medium
Pomegranate	1 medium
Prunes	¼ cup
Quince	1 medium
Raisins	¼ cup
Sapote†	1 medium
Tangerine†	1 medium
Watermelon	½ cup

THE HUMBLE LEGUMES

Until the 1990s, many Americans had tasted legumes only three ways: as baked beans, in minestrone soup, and in three-bean salad, that mélange of green beans, waxed beans, and kidney beans drowned in oil and vinegar. Then several trends converged, and legume cookery moved to the front burner. It's on the third level of the Power-Up Food Plan Pyramid.

First, an onslaught of nutrition research confirmed the unequaled healthfulness of legumes (or beans, if you prefer), with protein, fiber, iron, and the B vitamins heading the list. Dietary fat? Zilch, with one exception: soybeans. Soybeans have become the most celebrated legume, chiefly through the foods made from them, such as tofu, tempeh, soymilk, miso, and texturized vegetable protein. Numerous studies have suggested that eating soy regularly may fend off cancer and heart disease.

Among the most intriguing findings: As natural storehouses of the B vitamin folic acid, legumes have a say in keeping down your body's level of homocysteine, an amino acid that some scientists believe is as risky at high levels as smoking. It may even be more damaging to your health than cholesterol.

Second, savvy marketers have pumped the public on the huge variety of tasty and unusual legumes and made them available in stores and by mail order. Among them are rattlesnake beans and adzukis, little Japanese treasures.

And, finally, celebrated chefs like Mark Miller at the renowned Coyote Cafe in Sante Fe have created exquisite legume-studded dishes that wow their patrons. Other chefs have joined their lead. The stodgiest women's magazines have chimed in, serving up recipes for black bean soup and marinated white beans with herbs.

Why was this flavorful vegetarian staple ignored by the masses until recently? Probably cooks didn't have many recipes for legumes, pooh-poohed their peasantry, and mistakenly believed that they're difficult to prepare. Not so. Cooking from scratch is just a matter of soaking and simmering. If that's too much trouble, buy canned. Just rinse before using, because the liquid in canned beans is usually salty.

Though hundreds of legume varieties are available, here are the most common:

Black beans: These small, oval-shaped legumes have a robust flavor and work well with strong herbs and spices. A must in Cuban cooking. Also known as black turtle beans.

Black-eyed peas: Creamy white with a black spot or "eye," these legumes have a fresh flavor and are popular in Southern cooking.

Chickpeas: These round, golden legumes have a nutty flavor. A favorite in Mediterranean dishes, especially falafel. Also called garbanzo beans.

Great northern beans: Subtlety flavored, these white legumes work well in soups and as dips and sandwich spreads.

Kidney beans: Related to red beans, which are smaller and

rounder than kidney beans, these legumes show up in salads, chili, and Hispanic dishes.

Lentils: Available in green, brown, and red varieties, these small, disk-shaped legumes have an earthy flavor. They're a favorite in soup but also appear in pilafs and ethnic dishes.

Lima beans: The smaller ones taste somewhat sweet. The larger ones, also called butter beans, are "beanier." Either works well in a variety of dishes.

Navy beans: The choice for baked beans, these legumes look like miniature great northern beans.

Pinto beans: Integral to Hispanic cooking, these pinkish legumes have a mild flavor and a creamy texture when cooked.

Soybeans: The current world champ in nutrition, these legumes taste bland and take a long time to cook. Most popular are soybean spinoffs, including tofu, tempeh, miso, soymilk, and texturized vegetable protein (usually called TVP).

Split peas: Earthy yet sweet, split peas make a fantastic soup. They're not common in other dishes because they cook up very soft.

Interested in the exotics? Request a catalog from mail-order companies specializing in legumes. Two are the Bean Bag (800-845-2326) and Dean and Deluca (800-221-7714).

Each serving of legumes equals one selection in the Power-Up Food Plan. A serving provides about 125 calories, 20 grams of carbohydrates, 9 grams of protein, a negligible amount of fat (except for soybeans), no cholesterol, and 10 grams of fiber.

ITEM	SERVING SIZE
Legumes, any type	½ cup, cooked
Miso	¼ cup
Soymilk	1 cup
Tempeh	½ cup
Tofu, firm	½ cup

CRAZY ABOUT NUTS

I used to avoid nuts, because I believed they were little more than fat. But after doing some research, I'm happy to admit I was wrong.

Though mostly fat (with the exception of water chestnuts, which have only 15 percent of calories from fat), nuts and seeds generally are good sources of zinc, magnesium, manganese, and folic acid. Sunflower seeds chime in with vitamin B_6. Peanuts and hazelnuts contribute boron. Almonds, filberts, walnuts, and nut oils have lots of vitamin E. Brazil nuts, pine nuts, and tahini (ground sesame seeds) serve up vitamin B_1. Peanuts, pecans, and sunflower seeds offer pantothenic acid.

Surprisingly, the common walnut stands alone with special health honor. It teems with heart-healthy omega-3 fatty acids.

As mentioned, adequate amounts of these vitamins and minerals are crucial to the body's ability to manufacture neurotransmitters and, in turn, power up your mind, mood, and body. A couple of the nuts—peanuts and pecans—even contain the precursor to one of your brain's memory-managing neurotransmitters, acetylcholine. So next time you're faced with the decision to get nutty, why not do it?

Another delicious reason to eat nuts and seeds: They add a range of flavors and textures to your meals.

Each serving of nuts or seeds equals one selection in the Power-Up Food Plan. A serving provides about 175 calories, 6 grams of carbohydrates, 6 grams of protein, 14 grams of fat, no cholesterol, and less than 1 gram of fiber.

ITEM	SERVING SIZE
Nuts, most types	1 ounce or 2 tablespoons
Chestnuts	⅓ cup
Coconut, dried	¼ cup
Gingko nuts	⅓ cup
Seeds, any type	1 ounce or 2 tablespoons

THE BEST DAIRY FOODS

You've probably seen the milk mustache advertisements. It seems that everyone from Isabella Rossellini to Patrick Ewing has a white stripe under the nose. The message: Drink milk just like your favorite celebrity and you'll be successful and beautiful too.

Dairy foods do have a few health advantages—calcium and melatonin, to name two. Yet some are better for you than others.

The best: skim milk (no fat, 4 milligrams of cholesterol, about 300 milligrams of calcium per eight-ounce glass, and fortified with vitamins A and D) and nonfat or low-fat plain yogurt (minimal fat, 4 milligrams of cholesterol, about 450 milligrams of calcium per eight ounces).

Also respectable choices: low-fat cottage cheese (about 2 grams of fat, 10 milligrams of cholesterol, and 138 milligrams of calcium in one cup) and buttermilk (minimal fat, 9 milligrams of cholesterol, and about 285 milligrams of calcium per eight-ounce glass).

The worst: eggnog (19 grams of fat, 149 milligrams of cholesterol, 330 milligrams of calcium, and lots of refined sugar in an eight-ounce glass), milkshake (9 grams of fat, 35 milligrams of cholesterol, 290 milligrams of calcium, and lots of refined sugar in an eight-ounce glass), and full-fat cheese (about 9 grams of fat, 30 milligrams of cholesterol, and nearly 200 milligrams of calcium in an ounce).

Also poor choices: cream cheese (10 grams of fat, 30 milligrams of cholesterol, and 23 milligrams of calcium in two tablespoons), whole-milk ricotta cheese (16 grams of fat, 63 milligrams of cholesterol, and 257 milligrams of calcium in one-half cup), and whole milk (8 grams of fat, 35 milligrams of cholesterol, and 290 milligrams of calcium per eight-ounce glass).

The in-betweeners: low-fat cheese (about 4 grams of fat, 15 milligrams of cholesterol, and 200 milligrams of calcium in an ounce), fruited yogurt (about 3 grams of fat, 10 milligrams of cholesterol, 315 milligrams of calcium, and lots of refined sugar), creamed cottage cheese (10 grams of fat, 30 milligrams of cholesterol, and 126 milligrams of calcium in a cup), and part-skim ricotta cheese (9 grams of fat, 38 milligrams of cholesterol, and 337 milligrams of calcium in one-half cup).

All of these dairy foods have ample amounts of vitamin B_{12}, crucial to your nervous system and found reliably only in animal foods and fortified foods like some cereals and soy products. Check labels. Dairy foods contain no fiber.

Each serving of dairy foods equals one selection in the Power-Up Food Plan.

CALCIUM MINUS THE COW

Dairy products aren't the only foods rich in calcium. Here are some high-calcium plant sources.

Collards, 1 cup cooked: 358 milligrams (mg)
Figs, 10 dried: 269mg
Tofu, firm, made with calcium salts, ½ cup: 258mg
Spinach, 1 cup cooked: 244mg
Broccoli, 1 cup cooked: 178mg
Okra, 1 cup cooked: 176mg
Amaranth, ½ cup cooked: 138mg
Blackstrap molasses, 1 tablespoon: 137mg
Tempeh (a soyfood), ½ cup: 77mg
Great northern beans, ½ cup cooked: 65mg
Navy beans, ½ cup cooked: 64mg
Pinto beans, ½ cup cooked: 45mg

It's assumed that the selection is nonfat or low-fat. A low-fat serving provides about 100 calories, 12 grams of carbohydrates, 9 grams of protein, and 0 to 4 grams of fat.

(*) indicates a high-fat choice.

ITEM	SERVING SIZE
Buttermilk	1 cup
Cheese:	
Nonfat or low-fat	1 ounce
Whole*	1 ounce
Cottage cheese:	
Low-fat	¾ cup
Creamed*	¾ cup

ITEM	SERVING SIZE
Cream cheese:	
Nonfat	2 tablespoons
Low-fat*	2 tablespoons
Regular	2 tablespoons
Milk:	
Evaporated nonfat milk	½ cup
Nonfat	1 cup
Low-fat or whole*	1 cup
Ricotta cheese:	
Low-fat	⅓ cup
Part-skim*	⅓ cup
Whole*	⅓ cup
Yogurt:	
Nonfat or low-fat	1 cup
Whole*	1 cup

EGGS AND MEAT DE-EMPHASIZED

The gruesome twosome?

That's the suggestion of many research studies indicting eggs and meat for their cholesterol and saturated fat contents and their link to bacterial-related diseases. But press releases from the egg and meat industries proclaim their healthfulness and have the USDA's Food Guide Pyramid to back them up. Take a look at it and what do you see?—two to three servings of meat and/or eggs each and every day.

It's no wonder people are confused about what to eat.

The Ultimate version of my Power-Up Food Plan lets you eat

one serving, or no servings, of foods in the egg and meat family. Here's why.

A wealth of research studies show that a largely vegetarian diet is the healthiest. The various studies include many populations: the Chinese, the Okinawans, the Greeks, the Californian Seventh-Day Adventists (who belong to a Protestant denomination that praises the vegetarian diet), as well as African tribes and various other peoples.

The overall conclusion: The less meat and fewer eggs eaten, the greater health. Not only the vegetarians, but also those who eat a very small amount of meat or eggs enjoy excellent health.

In addition, the protein in meats is a major supplier of the amino acid homocysteine, which is dangerous in quantity. The body gets homocysteine from methionine, another amino acid, present in animal foods. Chomp into a roast beef sandwich or even a slice of lean turkey breast and your homocysteine levels go up.

In a landmark study in 1997, researchers found that homocysteine levels of their study's heart patients predicted with amazing accuracy who would die of a heart attack. Those with high levels were three to six times more likely to die than those with low levels.

Though I made the vegetarian choice fourteen years ago with no regrets, I know many people who are almost vegetarian and seem healthy too. And so combining the research conclusions with my experience—both personal and in my wellness counseling—I settled on zero to one daily serving of the egg and meat family.

Each serving of eggs or meat equals one selection in the Power-Up Food Plan. A serving provides about 150 calories, 20 grams of protein, and up to 20 grams of fat, 100 milligrams of cholesterol (but 275 milligrams for one egg), and no fiber. These foods are also high in iron, zinc, and the B vitamins.

Three ounces of meat is equal in size to a deck of cards.

An ounce of luncheon meat is equal to one slice.

ITEM	SERVING SIZE
Beef:	
Flank, round, top round roast, and other lean cuts	3 ounces
Ground, porterhouse, ribs, and other fatty cuts	2 ounces
Eggs	2 eggs
Fish and seafood	3 ounces
Luncheon meats	1 ounce
Pork	3 ounces
Poultry, without skin	3 ounces

BETTER FATS, SWEETER SWEETS

See if you can solve this riddle:

Americans are eating less fat (about 34 percent of total calories, down from 40 percent in a few short years) and yet we keep getting fatter. One-third of American adults are obese, up from one-quarter. How so?

The answer: Though the fat percentage is dropping, we're piling our plates with calories, especially high-sugar, nonfat items. Call it the SnackWell's Syndrome.

The truth is, oodles of calories pack most nonfat and low-fat foods, while the equation for gaining or losing body fat remains the same. Generally speaking,

If calories consumed equal calories burned, then body weight stays constant.

But if calories consumed are greater than calories burned, then either eat less or exercise more to lose excess pounds— or go on a shopping spree for larger clothes.

The smartest choice is to eat healthy portions of fat and sugar. In excess, either can sabotage the Power-Up Food Plan.

The problem with fat seems obvious. It's weighty food, literally. A gram of fat has nine calories, or more than twice as much as a gram of either carbos or protein. Fat also slips easily into fat stores. And when your body digests fat, it burns only three out of every one hundred calories of fat, so ninety-seven are primed for storage.

Higher fat diets (containing over 25 percent of total calories from fat) are also linked to killer diseases, including some cancers, heart disease, stroke, and obesity.

The type of fat you eat matters too.

The worst are trans fatty acids and saturated fats. Put on your detective garb to detect the deadly trans fats; they don't show up on nutrition labels. Rather, turn to a product's ingredient list for phrases like "partially hydrogenated soybean oil." The word "hydrogenated" is the tipoff. When you see it, assume that trans fats lurk inside the product in question.

As for saturated fats, which can lead to clogged arteries and a compromised immune system, they appear not only in animal foods like meat, dairy, and eggs but also a selected group of vegetables, namely coconut and palm kernel oils. Keep saturated fats and trans fats to a minimum, no more than 7 percent of the total calories in your diet.

That's about 140 calories, or about 15 grams of saturated fats or trans fats, for a person averaging 2,000 total calories a day. Fifteen grams equal about two ounces of cheddar cheese, a cup of vanilla soft-serve ice cream, or two tablespoons of butter.

The better fats are olive, safflower, and canola oils in modest amounts. For instance, sauté vegetables in a teaspoon of oil. If the pan gets dry, add wine or vegetable stock a tablespoon or two at a time. Replace the butter in a cookie recipe with fat-reduced margarine (some say "no trans fats" on the package), using about three-quarters of the amount called for. You'll find more fat-cutting ideas in the recipe section. While everyone talks about trimming fat, most could care less about sugar. But sugar and the sweets made from it can be lemon-sour to your body. (See "A Too Sweet Problem," page 28, for details.)

Face it, sugar lovers: A high-carbo diet that's low in fiber could set you up for serious illness as well as fuzzy thinking, mood swings, and poor energy.

Not only that, sugar replaces the nutritious foods you could be feasting on. When you eat poorly, you think poorly, feel poorly, and perform poorly.

The flip side is true too.

If you want to think your best . . .
If you want to feel your best . . .   *. . . Eat Your Best!*
If you want to perform your best . . .

The take-to-the-kitchen message: Go easy on fat and sugar, and you'll look, feel, and think great.

By the way, there is no recommended number of servings of fat or sweets on the Power-Up Food Plan, but here's a guideline: Get about 20 to 25 percent of your total calories from fat and no more than 10 percent of your total calories from refined sugar.

The list below gives you an idea of the fat in selected foods.

THE FAT-GRAM COUNTER

ITEM	SERVING SIZE	FAT
Butter	1 tablespoon	12.3g
Cheese:	1 ounce	
cheddar		9.8g
mozzarella		4.5g
soy		5.0g
Chocolate chips	¼ cup	12.2g
Croissant	1 medium	12.0g
Egg	1 egg	5.6g
Fruit, all	normal portion	less than 1g
Grains	normal portion	about 1g

ITEM	SERVING SIZE	FAT
Legumes:	½ cup cooked	
most		less than 1g
chickpeas		2.2g
soybeans		5.1g
Margarine:	1 tablespoon	
reduced fat		6.0g
regular		12.0g
Milk:	1 cup	
skim		less than 1g
2-percent		4.7g
whole		8.0g
Nuts	1 ounce	12 to 14g
Oil, all types	1 tablespoon	13.6g
Salad dressing:	1 tablespoon	
reduced fat		1.5g
regular		6 to 8g
Seeds	1 ounce	12 to 14g
Tofu:	½ cup	
firm		11.0g
soft		6.0g
reduced fat		4.0g
Tortilla, flour	1 large	3.8g
Vegetables:		
all except olives and avocado	normal portion	less than 1g
avocado	1 medium	30.0g
olives	4 large	8.0g
Yogurt, low-fat	1 cup	2.5g

THE SNEAKY SUGAR SOIREE

A problem with refined sugar, beyond the obvious, is that it can be difficult to detect. Just grab any packaged food you have on hand and turn to the label's "Nutrition Facts."

First let's check milk. On the label, it states that a one-cup serving has eleven grams of sugar, but I know that no sugar has been added to the milk. Rather, this sugar is lactose, a naturally occurring simple carbo. It should not be counted as a refined sugar on the Power-Up Food Plan.

Trickier to figure out is low-sugar red raspberry preserves. A one-tablespoon serving has five grams of sugar. Some is fructose, a naturally occurring sugar in raspberries, and some is refined sugar.

How do I know? I checked the ingredient list. The second ingredient listed is sugar, followed by water, fruit pectin, and a few other ingredients. But I still do not know how many of the five grams of sugar listed in the Nutrition Facts is refined.

Your best bet in determining the amount of refined sugar is a two-step method:

First, ask yourself whether the food contains naturally occurring sugars like lactose in milk, fructose in most fruits, or glucose in some fruits like grapes, figs, and dates. If it contains naturally occurring sugars, then assume that at least some, and possibly all, of the "sugars" are not refined.

Second, look at the product's ingredient list. If you spot high fructose corn syrup, corn syrup, dextrose, sucrose, and/or other sweeteners, then it contains refined sugar. And if one of these words is among the first three ingredients or there are two or more on the list, the product probably has a load of refined sugar. (Ingredients are listed in order of amount.) Remember to keep your consumption of products that are filled with refined sugars to a healthy minimum.

Another example is my nine-year-old's favorite store-bought granola bars. I scan down to the "total carbohydrate" line of the Nutrition Facts and note "sugars" at ten grams per serving.

The ingredient list includes these words: brown sugar, honey, corn syrup, sugar, high fructose corn syrup, sorbitol, and molasses. They spell refined sugar. In estimating the number of grams of refined sugar, I choose nine because of the obvious sugary status of Laura's granola bars and I start thinking about developing my own less-sugar-but-still-yummy recipe. Until the Nutrition Facts are improved to distinguish between refined and naturally occurring sugars, an estimation is the best anyone can do.

Let me make my case even stronger.

In front of me is a can of pineapple chunks in pineapple juice. The ingredients listed are pineapple, pineapple juice, water, and clarified pineapple juice concentrate but no refined sugar of any type. And yet the Nutrition Facts list sugars at thirteen grams per serving, even higher than the granola bars.

So should I pick the granola bars over pineapple chunks for a healthy snack? No way. All of the sugar in the pineapple chunks are naturally occurring, not refined. I may eat my sweet pineapple treat (and not count them toward my allotment of refined sugar) in true power-eating style:

With gusto!

Get Up and Power-cise

My friend Pam is a double-take woman. You take one look at her and, whether you're a man or a woman, you sneak a second peek. Her looks are that good. Ocean-blue eyes, long, sandy hair, a smile that could earn her a spot on a toothpaste commercial, a great physique. She's genuinely nice, self-confident, and *real* too.

It's a combination I rarely see. And, I confess, Pam inspires me.

A living picture of a power-up exerciser, she taps and jazz-dances alongside her dance students for twelve or so hours each week, and she walks, cycles, or dances a few more times a week, just for herself.

It's not fear of cancer that moves this mother of two school-aged kids. No, it's something far simpler: an exercise high.

"Sometimes I get to where I feel down and blobby," Pam admits. "But once I gear up and do something physical, I feel uplifted. I feel better mentally. Exercising keeps me motivated, organized, and moving forward." Pam says dancing has alleviated cold symptoms more times than she can count.

Her experience reads like a medical journal detailing the latest research on exercise and improved thinking, better mood, and peak physical performance. The bottom line: Physical activity greatly determines your level of health (mind, mood, body, and spirit)—today and tomorrow, with emphasis on today.

Let's be honest. The reason Pam or I or anyone bothers to exercise isn't really to avoid killer diseases that may never kill us. We want immediate payoffs. Let it be said, however, that a 1996 report from the U.S. Surgeon General cited regular activity as the best way to sashay past chronic illness like heart disease and many types of cancer—and feel happier too.

Exercise can almost instantly boost your mood, reduce anxiety, improve concentration, create calm, and rev up your metabolism. Other benefits may take a little longer to see (say, a few weeks—less if you're already in good physical shape), including higher energy, improved sleep, a more positive self-image, sustained body fat loss, and better memory.

Now for some surprises about exercise:

- More isn't necessarily better.
- Pain is *not* gain.
- Huffing and puffing is bad for your health.

Truly, top exercise physiologists have discovered that the ability to run a marathon or clean-and-jerk a few hundred pounds fails as a benchmark of enviable physicality. Chances are, the health of many marathoners and gym rats leaves much to be desired. Rather, the power-up exerciser, or power-ciser, scores top marks.

So who are these power-cisers?

Let's paint a portrait.

They move. Movement is natural to them, as flight is to an eagle or pouncing is to a snow leopard. They give it little thought. They just move. They may not even call it exercise. And they never call it difficult.

They move many ways: pumping their hearts, strengthening their muscles (from the trapezoids clear down to the calves), and stretching their tendons, ligaments, and muscles all over their bodies.

Like Pam, they delight in the sheer pleasure of movement and its feel-good sensations, thanks to the endorphins that soothe their bodies, lift their spirits, and keep them coming back for more.

The word *endorphin* literally means "endogenous morphine," or "morphine from within." At birth, you came packaged with this neurotransmitter for a reason. The endorphins help you tolerate pain, physical and emotional. One example is childbirth. During this miracle, the endorphins are released at two hundred times their normal levels. You might debate—particularly if you're a woman who has borne a child or her coach, who witnessed the contortions of pain—whether Mother Nature could have done a better job.

Before you're tempted to criticize, just imagine childbirth—or a broken leg or a ruptured appendix or a bullet wound—without the endorphins. I hope a waterfall of thanksgiving showers you instead.

HOW EXERCISE CURBS CRAVINGS

As you know, people who exercise are more likely to maintain a healthy weight than nonexercisers. But burning extra calories during badminton, basketball, or dancing isn't the only reason for this well-documented conclusion.

Studies suggest exercisers are also less likely to pig out on their craved foods because they have fewer cravings.

Remember, biological food cravings are good. They tell you that you need a specific nutrient or an alteration in your brain chemistry. You only need a small amount of food to fulfill a biological food craving.

The problem is, your craved goodie may taste so good, so soothing, so right, that you may overeat it. If you overeat, you probably are eating for emotional reasons.

A solution: exercise.

The right type encourages an endorphin release. The endorphins are the neurotransmitters that elicit a sense of subtle ecstasy. Your endorphins are your own private stash of morphine that you can access through exercise. Though research continues, the endorphin release is thought to be at the heart of reduced food cravings.

In her book, *Why Women Need Chocolate*, Debra Waterhouse reports 39 percent fewer fat cravings, 32 percent fewer chocolate cravings, and 22 percent fewer sugar cravings among the women she surveyed who exercised regularly.

So which exercise gives you an endorphin high? Any exercise that creates a beneficial stress in your muscles, joints, and cardiovascular system.

Physical stress is the key, because the endorphins are released as an analgesic, or painkiller. Without physical stress, the body won't release them. Unless you're out of shape, a twenty-minute walk probably isn't stressful enough for your body to start feeling sorry for you and give you a boost of endorphins.

Rather, the best exercise for you must be of sufficient duration and intensity. You'll need to push yourself a bit, without going overboard. If you exercise too long and too hard your first day out, you may call it quits.

For an ongoing curb of cravings, simply pick a favorite exercise and a reasonable but challenging intensity and duration. For instance, if you're a walker who usually covers two miles in thirty minutes, try three miles in forty minutes. If you prefer a team sport like basketball, and usually play two back-to-back full-court games, go for three or four full-court games. Like to swim? Increase your laps by a third or more.

You'll notice at least two things:

First, as your body gets used to the greater intensity and duration of exercise, you'll need to push yourself a bit more to get an endorphin boost.

Second, as the endorphins send their feel-good messages, you'll wave good-bye to many food cravings.

Likewise, the endorphins figure in mightily to exercise. Exercise stresses your body. The stress prompts the pituitary gland to say, "Hey, it's time for some endorphins." With their release, you get high. Admit it, you inhaled deeply, didn't you?

It's a wonderfully clean high. While endorphins are chemically similar to the pain reliever morphine, although about two hundred times more potent, you don't become red-eyed, dazed, and desperate like a hard-core drug addict. To the contrary, like Pam, you think with greater acuity, you feel contented and relaxed, you improve your strength and endurance, you charge your immune system and increase your longevity, and you want more, more, more.

Yes, it's possible to lean on exercise like a crutch. You can escape within it, hide behind it, and live for it and little else. Do so and you're not—repeat, not—a power-ciser.

On the flip side shuffle most Americans. Statistics indicate that 60 percent of Americans rarely break a sweat. It's easy to see why. We've got cars, escalators, TV remote controls, and every other gadget to make our lives easier—in other words, less active. Remember the days before electric can openers? You actually had to wrestle with a manual one to open a can of soup.

As bad as our sloth is, it's the rush-rush mentality that infects Americans like a bubonic plague and fells many of us. In the effort to buy bigger houses, acquire more credit cards, drive fancier cars, and on and on and on, we work longer hours, get stressed out, and lose a precious gift: our true selves.

Back to getting up and power-cising.

In the pages to come, you'll find out why power-cising is such an important companion to the Power-Up Food Plan. It energizes, makes you smarter, enhances your mood, charges up your immunity, and brings down your weight. To put power-cising into practice, you'll see three doable plans for various fitness levels and interests at the end of this chapter.

■ STEP UP TO HIGH ENERGY ■

Exercise is explosive, ushering forth energy that you can harness and use to power up your mind, mood, and body. We'll look at these three in turn, in a few moments.

First, let's see how exercise makes energy.

Exercise tones muscles, and toned muscles lead to improved body efficiency. And improved efficiency makes every movement easier and more graceful, from lifting a pen and carrying a baby to jogging a mile and climbing Mount Everest.

The exercise path to a fit cardiovascular system is **aerobic** activity. In other words, exercise that increases your heart rate strengthens your heart, which is busy delivering oxygen to your hungry muscles to meet their working demands. Ample oxygen to your muscles almost guarantees stepped-up pep.

I say "almost" because your body's muscle tissue needs a tune-up too. If your muscles are out of shape, they barely know what to do with the extra oxygen. Blame it on mitochondria, if you must. The muscle tissue of unfit people contains too few mitochondria, the microscopic "brains" of body cells, which help turn fuel from food into energy.

The exercise path to fit muscles is **strength-training.** Barbells, dumbbells, oversized rubber bands, Nautilus machines, your own body weight—all of these can help build muscle. There are more reasons than I can count to muscle up, but the foremost is increased energy. As you build muscle, ordinary activities, like carrying the groceries, require less effort.

Research indicates that regular physical activity, both aerobic and strength-training, improves body efficiency and, in turn, boosts energy. In one study, the resting heart rates of middle-aged men dropped from an average of seventy-two beats per minute to fifty-five after working out regularly for three months.

Body efficiency figures into my new energy equation: $E = ep^2$, with e standing for body efficiency, p for power-eating, and E for super energy. When exercise-induced body efficiency combines with power-eating (eating the right foods at the right times in the right combinations), you will feel your energy zoom exponentially.

Here's a real-life example: I'm under a tight deadline to finish a book and so I work late into the night. Knowing what I do about power-eating, I stay away from carbos and instead eat a protein-rich, low-fat snack like yogurt.

The amino acid tyrosine in protein blocks tryptophan, an amino acid known to turn on the "comforting" neurotransmitter serotonin that could fuzz my brain, because I'm already tired. (If I were anxious, the extra serotonin would create calm.) So I remain energized, but not as much as I'd like.

What can I do to boost my energy?

You guessed it: exercise. Almost any physical activity will do—scrubbing the bathroom tile with a toothbrush, for instance—but I select jumping up and down on a minitrampoline in my office. Ten minutes of bouncing to the beat have left me relaxed, feeling good, and wide awake. I'm poised to click away at my keyboard for another hour or two.

There are at least two other important ways that exercise gives you zip. One is its psychological benefits. The other is the endorphin high.

Hundreds, perhaps thousands, of studies have shown that exercise lessens depression, anxiety, and stress—all of which steal energy. You might remember from chapter 3 that energy is one of the two main components of mood. The other is calm. Calm-energy is the very definition of good mood. Admittedly depression, anxiety, and stress can rear their ugly heads time and again. That's why lackadaisical exercise is a loser. Regular exercise is best, but never hard or boring or a pain.

It can get you high, too. The endorphin high is not for marathoners only. Any regular Jo can experience it if she stresses her muscles hard enough and long enough.

Owen Anderson, Ph.D., related this tale in *Runner's World:*

"My brother started first—running slowly around the curve of the track. I followed. We moved lethargically for a couple of laps but gradually picked up the pace and finished our inaugural mile in 7:25.

"As I tried to keep pace, my lungs heaved, and sweat streamed down my legs into my Chuck Taylor All-Stars. A sharp pain speared the left side of my abdomen, and each rapid, forceful heartbeat transformed my head into a booming bass drum. This was the most agonizing thing I had ever done. Somehow, we stumbled through three miles . . . and collapsed onto the infield.

"My body's agony turned into warm relaxation. The pain eased, and I felt more at peace than I had ever been before. I didn't realize it then, but I was experiencing my first of many 'runner's highs.' "

As mentioned, you can get high without heaving or booming or collapsing. While stress—physical or emotional—triggers the release of energizing endorphins, scientist Atko Viro, Ph.D., has found that exercising at about 75 percent of your maximum heart rate can do the trick. The research on the duration of exercise for endorphin release is mixed, most likely due to individual differences.

At least one thing's for sure: Jogging, cycling, swimming, dancing, and similar activities, provided they're of sufficient intensity and duration, will produce endorphins. Numbers aside, you can be confident you're releasing endorphins when suddenly you experience a burst of new physical energy and feel like you could keep going for hours, when your senses become heightened (colors seem brighter, for instance), and/or when you have creative notions and inspiring ideas.

You can count on a brain boost too.

■ MIND: SMARTENING UP ■

As incredible as it seems, mounting evidence suggests that exercise can help you think clearer, concentrate better, memorize easier, and, in general, delight in greater intellectual prowess. Exercise is no magic elixir, however. If that were so, relatively smart people like Michael Jordan ought to be extraordinary geniuses by now. But M. J.'s not a card-carrying Mensa member—yet. (Believe me, my husband, the slam-dunking sports encyclopedia, would have told me.)

Though physical activity in itself won't make you a genius, it can and does improve thinking abilities. How?

In two words, blood flow.

When your heart's pumping hard, the blood flow to your brain increases, bathing it in oxygen and glucose ("blood sugar"). Your brain needs thirty times more blood than other organs. The more it has, the greater your ability to think well.

In one study, participants took various tests measuring aspects of intelligence, including verbal fluency and perceptiveness, before and after a twenty-six day regimen of daily walks and an almost vegetarian diet. These thirty-one volunteers each suffered a chronic illness of some sort—heart disease, diabetes, or arthritis—and the average age of the group was sixty. Their "after" scores were significantly higher.

A good workout can blow out the mental cobwebs another way. Some researchers say that repetitive motions like jogging, brisk walking, and swimming shut down the left side of the brain. The left side is responsible for logical and analytical thought.

The brain's activity shifts mainly to the right side, which is associated with abstract and creative thinking. Left-brain, right-brain proponents say this shift explains the bright, creative thoughts that seem to come out of nowhere during a jog.

Other studies have looked at exercise and memory, a brain function that often wanes as we age. But it doesn't have to.

In addition to power-eating (especially high-choline foods like eggs, soy foods, and wheat germ) and playing mind games (see "Checkers, Anyone?" page 136), exercise makes a big difference in your ability to remember well.

In a study of adults in their forties, one group walked and jogged regularly for ten weeks. The other group remained sedentary. The exercisers easily outperformed their slothful counterparts in a test of numbers that both groups had been asked to memorize. Another study found that older adults who took up brisk walking for four months, while a control group barely moved a muscle, improved in six out of eight mental ability tests, including short-term memory. The sedentary people showed no improvement.

■ MOOD: THE BIG LIFT ■

A routine prescription for people with mild to severe mood disorders like depression and anxiety is exercise. Regular physical activity of any sort can lift sagging spirits, especially if you have a minor case of the blues, in a number of ways.

Edmund J. Bourne, Ph.D., lists them in his award-winning *Anxiety and Phobia Workbook:*

- reduced tension in the muscles, which is largely responsible for your feeling "uptight" and "in knots"
- quicker metabolism of excess adrenaline, a stress hormone that can keep you in a state of arousal, leading to anxiety
- a discharge of pent-up frustration, which can aggravate depression, the blues, and anxiety
- increase in the endorphins, opiates (painkillers) produced by the body, which increase your sense of well-being

Ironically, the discovery of the mind-body link began with heart patients, not bad-mood complainers. Back in the early

1970s, cardiologists noticed that patients who were exercising to strengthen their damaged hearts were also experiencing dramatic psychological improvements. Since then, hundreds of studies have examined the correlation.

A watershed report by the National Institutes of Mental Health in 1984 trumpeted the mood-boosting effect of exercise. Among the findings: Regular exercise lowers readings on stress indicators, including resting heart rate, neuromuscular tension, and some stress hormone levels. People who work out year after year also are less likely to develop serious mental-health problems. That's true for both genders and all ages.

Thank your endorphins again.

Runners call the marked jump of endorphins in their body chemistry a "high." Mountain bikers call it "bliss." Swimmers call it "sweet." Those who have mild to severe mood disorders or who are just battling the blues say it's medicine.

Studies show that endorphin levels can increase by as much as five times the resting amount after twelve minutes of vigorous exercise, and they continue to circulate at high levels for up to thirty minutes.

Along with the endorphins, the neurotransmitter norepinephrine gets a boost during exercise. Mental-health experts have long known that depressed patients often lack an ample supply of norepinephrine, so it came as no surprise when researchers found that regular exercisers with high norepinephrine levels tend to be happier and less stressed.

To get the biggest mood boost, think moderation. Research shows that exercisers who work hard enough to break a sweat but who stay within comfortable limits are the happiest. One study, for instance, compared marathoners, 10k runners, and beginners. The 10k-ers as a whole scored lowest on all the measures of bad mood.

If you're a beginner, you may not reap good-mood benefits for a couple of weeks, because you may have muscle soreness and a bit of trouble getting used to an exercise routine.

So hang in there and feel your spirits soar.

P.S. You can become fitter without pumping up to the levels I described above. Exercise physiologists are now saying that any physical activity—mowing the lawn, kicking around the soccer ball with the kids, mopping the floors—offers health benefits. All you need is thirty minutes, and not all at once: a little here, a little there, throughout the day. There's no need to figure your heart rate either.

Supporting the advocates of exercise-lite is a study at the Cooper Aerobics Research Institute, in which about 120 volunteers followed the standard gym recommendations and another 120 volunteers tried exercise-lite. Both groups on average reduced their blood pressure by eight points, lowered total cholesterol, and gained about the same amount of muscle and dropped about the same amount of fat.

What about boosting endorphins while exercising-lite?

While more research is needed, I wouldn't bet on it. The preponderance of evidence points to the need of stressing muscles for the release of the endorphins. Exercise-lite seems too lite to qualify.

▪ BODY I: REV UP YOUR IMMUNITY ▪

Medical science has yet to find the cure for the common cold, but there's new evidence on how to avoid it: Get up and go.

Moderate exercise is proving itself as an effective shot in the arm to your immune system. It appears that within minutes of beginning a workout, your white blood cells, which gobble up nasty germs, increase in number. The count decreases to normal levels within a few hours. However, the temporary boost seems to wipe out intruders and keep them at bay all day long.

It makes sense, then, that exercisers have fewer bouts with colds and flus than do their sedentary peers. In a study of women in their thirties, one group walked briskly for forty-five minutes a day, five days a week, and they were sick with colds and flus an average of five days over a fifteen-week period during peak cold season. The sedentary group were sick twice as many days.

Another study with women in their sixties, seventies, and eighties found similar results. Half of the women walked thirty-seven minutes a day, five days a week, for twelve weeks; the others remained inactive. Fifty percent of the nonexercisers caught colds during the study, while only 21 percent of the walkers did.

More encouragement: The women who had been dedicated exercisers prior to the study fared even better. Only 8 percent fell ill.

Moderate exercise does wonders for people with serious illness too. A study of HIV-infected patients showed that those who rode exercise bikes for forty-five minutes, three times a week, boosted their CD4 cell count, which is a vital measurement of health in AIDS patients.

Another study looked at rheumatoid arthritis sufferers and found that lifting weights at 80 percent of their capacity slowed the muscle deterioration that occurs with this disease. Research also shows that weight-bearing exercise like jogging and weight-lifting increases and maintains bone density in both young and older people, helping to delay or minimize osteoporosis, a bone-thinning disease that often leads to fractures and sometimes death.

Only thirty years ago, most doctors advised patients with chronic illness to take it very easy and conserve their energy for healing. Nowadays, they prescribe moderate exercise.

Exercise has become such a standard recommendation to patients that nearly four hundred U.S. hospitals boast full-service gyms, including Olympic-size pools. At the Mayo Clinic, for instance, heart transplant patients typically get rooms outfitted with stationary bicycles, and within two days of surgery, they're peddling away.

The reason for the turnabout: Exercise can lengthen and improve the lives of people with everything from asthma and cancer to heart disease, lupus, and AIDS. It can free diabetics and hypertensives from their bottles of pills. It can allow nursing home patients to toss aside their canes.

That's what top scientists are saying, but a mystery remains: exactly how exercise works its magic.

They have some clues. A workout increases white blood cell count, triggers the release of certain hormones, and improves T-cell counts. While questions linger, scientists continue to marvel at an exercise-charged body's ability to fight disease, and, in turn, lengthen life. It's possible that an exerciser's immune system may even help stop the spread of cancer.

In *It's Better to Believe,* Kenneth Cooper, M.D., who probably knows more about fitness than anyone else, has this to say about exercise and longevity: "In my study of the human body, I've become convinced that most of us have the innate capacity to achieve vigorous lives well up into the upper end of the biblical longevity scale, or in excess of 100 years of age."

Cooper then serves up a method to figure out your "Real Age"—the functional or physiologic age at which

---

THE SEVENTH-INNING STRETCH

When someone says "exercise," what pops into your mind? Walking, spinning, dance, soccer, touch football, weight-lifting? How about stretching?

Limbering up as exercise is now gaining respect. It has a governmental stamp of approval in a set of guidelines known as Healthy People 2000, which encourages flexibility activities, such as stretching and yoga.

Of course, no fitness expert says to stretch *only.* But aerobic exercise and strength-training without flexibility is like a triangle with a missing point.

The bendability boom is not exactly backed by a plethora of studies. In fact, only a handful of well-designed ones exist. One of them found that people engaged in flexibility programs could turn their heads more easily, so they could drive better. It was funded by the AAA Foundation for Traffic Safety.

Another study compared stretching and flexibility exercises to a combination of walking, low-impact aerobics, and strength-training. For a year, about fifty previously sedentary people over age sixty-five limbered up, while another fifty of their peers took up the combo of muscling up the heart and body.

Researchers found that, as expected, the strength and endurance group improved their cardiovascular fitness, were burning more calories, and had stronger muscles. They also suffered more aches and pains, like bad backs. Those who did only stretching didn't strengthen their heart or muscles but they had far fewer aches and pains.

The take-to-the-gym message: You need aerobics, strength-training, *and* stretching in a well-rounded exercise program.

Stretching loosens up tense muscles. When a muscle is tight, it tells the brain to prepare for fight or flight. This causes the body to release stress hormones, which signal the muscles to tense up even more.

Here's where stretching comes in beautifully. Whether you bend down and reach toward your toes, like in grade school, or maneuver your body into the pretzel-like postures of yoga, stretching of any type extends hard-used muscles, bringing them back to their resting length. When you don't stretch, your muscles remain in a semicontracted state and they can get tired and sore.

That's an exercise expert's reason to stretch. Your reason may be simpler: It just feels so good.

your physical and mental capacities are currently operating. Figured in to your "Real Age," which often differs from your chronological age, are endurance, strength, flexibility, general health, and personal and family health history.

The sad truth is that the average American lives with a chronic illness that impairs life for about twelve years before death comes. But this depressing result isn't inevitable. You can enter your advanced years in a healthy state and greatly condense the time of limited function into a short period, immediately prior to death.

With an exercise-charged immune system, you can live long and well. You've heard what it takes.

So, in the words of a running-shoe giant, "Just do it."

▪ BODY II: A SLEEKER YOU ▪

When you exercise, a beautiful person comes to life. You!

I remember working with a woman I'll call Donna who discovered this for herself and hasn't stopped jumping up and down to a disco beat since. Prior to her exercise days, she was overweight and battle-weary. Her twenty-year marriage had ended in a messy divorce. With four kids and a full-time job, she barely had time to shower, let alone exercise.

Then it hit her, If she didn't nurture herself, she'd continue to feel rotten inside and out. So she made the first, bold step toward a better future. She signed on the dotted line and started exercising regularly—aerobics and strength-training three times a week—at a fitness club near her home.

As mentioned, aerobic exercise, such as brisk walking, jogging, rowing, and cross-country skiing, works the heart and lungs for a fit cardiovascular system. It makes your muscles stronger, but only to a point. Aerobics isn't as efficient as strength-training at building muscle. Plus, with a few exceptions, aerobic exercise does little to strengthen the upper body, where 65 percent of your muscles are. In contrast, strength-training is working out with some type of resistance to strengthen muscles and make them sleeker and healthier.

The reasons to muscle up are many, but here are the big three:

- Those who don't strength-train—and this includes aerobics enthusiasts—lose muscle mass at a rate of about one pound every two years. That amounts to a shocking loss of strength later in life. Things you may take for granted now—like opening a jar and walking around the block—become difficult, if not impossible.
- On a positive note, strength-trainers rev up their metabolism by adding muscle. Even at rest, muscle uses more calories than body fat does, so gaining extra muscle makes it easier to remain at a healthy weight throughout the decades.
- Strength-trainers look better too. As long as you're not toting a spare tire around your middle or saddlebags on your thighs, toned muscles mean sleek.

Though Donna didn't think she was weak when she joined the fitness club, she could handle very little weight at first—only ten pounds, for instance, on the butterfly machine, which strengthens the pectorals (chest muscles). But she stuck with it and reaped the benefits.

In just four months of thrice-weekly workouts, her body-fat percentage dropped from 33 percent to 24 percent. (The ideal body-fat percentage is 18 to 21 percent for women and 12 to 15 percent for men.) She had lost ten pounds and inches as well; her waist measured an enviable twenty-four inches.

Research underscores the sleek reason to combine aerobics and strength-training. In a study comparing a traditional aerobics program (cycling for thirty minutes three times a week) to a regimen of strength-training and aerobic exercise (cycling for fifteen minutes and using weight machines for fifteen minutes three times a week), the results were amazing.

After eight weeks of exercising, the cyclists lost four pounds of fat but gained no muscle, but the people who cycled and strength-trained lost ten pounds of fat and gained two pounds of muscle. The study involved seventy-two previously sedentary adults.

That's the beauty of exercising. The more you do it, the sleeker you get. Your body displays the inner changes that result from power-eating and power-cising.

Donna says, "Now there's this glow about me. I can't explain it, but I feel it. I see it."

▪ PICK YOUR POWER-CISE PLAN ▪

The best power-cise plan for you capitalizes on your strengths, improves your weaknesses, and uses your favorite types of exercise.

First, determine your current fitness level in endurance, strength, flexibility, and general health by answering the following questions:

1. *Endurance:* How fast can you walk a mile on a level surface? a) in less than 13 minutes b) in 14 or 15 minutes c) in more than 16 minutes
2. *Strength:* How many standard push-ups can you complete in one minute? a) at least 35 b) about 20 c) less than 15
3. *Flexibility:* While sitting on the floor, with legs straight in front of you and fingertips reaching beyond your heels, how far can you lean forward without bending your knees or bouncing? a) at least 4 inches beyond your heels (for women), at least 3

inches beyond your heels (for men) b) 3½ inches beyond your heels (for women), 2½ inches beyond your heels (for men) c) 3 inches or less beyond your heels (for women), 2 inches or less beyond your heels (for men)

4. *General health*: As determined by such medical tests as blood pressure, urinalysis, cholesterol and triglycerides, weight, PAP test, mammography, vision and hearing, and any other tests deemed important by your doctor, what is the state of your general health? a) excellent b) good c) poor

Next analyze your answers. The more *a* answers, the better your overall fitness. The more *c* answers, the more you have to improve.

Finally, select a power-cise plan based on your answers. The Novice is for those who marked one or two *c* answers to the first three questions and who are in good health. Did you choose mostly *b* answers and are in good health? The Apprentice is for you. If you marked *a* to each question (or just one *b* to the first three questions) and are in good or excellent health, you're probably ready for the Proficient.

Check with your doctor before starting any exercise program, particularly if you are in poor health.

THE NOVICE POWER-CISE PLAN

- Select a favorite from among the aerobic sports listed below, and start with two twenty-minute sessions a week. Work up to three twenty-minute sessions a week.
- Select a favorite from among the strength-training sports listed below, and do two ten-minute sessions a week, focusing on the major muscles: chest, back, shoulders, legs, biceps, triceps, and abdomen.
- Stretch gently for five to ten minutes after each exercise session.

THE APPRENTICE POWER-CISE PLAN

• Select a favorite from among the aerobic sports, and complete three thirty-minute sessions a week. Work up to three forty-minute sessions a week.
• Select a favorite from among the strength-training sports, and do two or three twenty-minute sessions a week, focusing on the major muscles: chest, back, shoulders, legs, biceps, triceps, and abdomen.
• Stretch gently for ten to fifteen minutes after each exercise session.

THE PROFICIENT POWER-CISE PLAN

• Select a favorite from among the aerobic sports; and complete three to five forty-minute sessions a week. Increase the duration and intensity of your exercise as desired.
• Select a favorite from among the strength-training sports, and complete three thirty- to forty-minute sessions a week, focusing on the major muscles: chest, back, shoulders, legs, biceps, triceps, and abdomen. You may strength-train daily if desired but rest an exercised muscle group for at least a day or two before working it out again.
• Choose a cross-training sport listed below, and spend at least a couple of hours having fun doing it each week.
• Stretch daily for at least ten to twenty minutes.

Remember, your favorite exercise is the best because you're most likely to stick with it and see fitness gains. You'll get the most gains from two- or three-times-a-week aerobic workouts, two- or three-times-a-week strength-training sessions, and daily stretching.

CHOOSE A SPORT

In the following lists of sports, circle the types you like best and cross out the ones you dislike.

▪ AEROBIC ▪

Aerobic dance (low-impact, high-impact, step)
Cycling (stationary)
Cycling (on road)
Dance (ballet, tap, jazz, square)
Jogging/running
Skiing (cross-country, outside, or simulator)
Swimming
Walking
Other: _____

▪ STRENGTH-TRAINING ▪

Calisthenics
Resistance rubber bands
Weight-lifting (machines, free weights like dumbbells)
Other: _____

▪ CROSS-TRAINING ▪

Baseball/softball
Basketball
Football
Gymnastics
Soccer
Volleyball
Other: _____

## nine

Power-Living for Life

Power-eating and power-cising: These can turn on the "everything clicks" switch in your brain, opening the door to clear thinking, enhanced mood, and peak physical performance. Aah, but there's more:

Power-living.

Power-living is choosing well among the hundreds—no, thousands—of options that dangle in front of you every day. Choose well and you achieve healthy balance. Choose poorly and face the ill consequences.

Should you stay at home full-time with your newborn or ride a lucrative career track? Take on an extra volunteer position or have much-needed quiet time? Stay up late to watch Clint Eastwood shoot the bad guys or get sleep? Make dinner or go to a fast-food drive-thru? Spend time in prayer or spend money at the mall?

Admittedly, this short list is all too black-and-white. Far more often our choices are shades of the rainbow, one blending into the next. Dozens of variables crisscross the possibilities so that one may not necessarily be right or even better. Sometimes we must choose between two heavenly options, or two evils—or, in truth, among many of them.

As mentioned, at the core of power-living is balance. Without it, we come unglued—or unbalanced, to use the popular term in this "age of anxiety." This unbalance leads to distress of every color, size, and shape: addiction, anxiety disorders, physical and mental disease, and, of course, pull-out-your-hair, punch-a-pillow stress and the rush-here, rush-there mentality the media have dubbed "hurry sickness." An apt description, I'd say.

Back a few years, as I wove between bodies on Fifty-second Street in New York City, a woman with "hurry sickness" plowed into me. No "excuse me" or "sorry." She just kept on walking, heels clicking, briefcase swinging, her eyes set squarely on the prize of success defined by human standards.

While a psychologist might tag the unbalanced with a diagnosis of "obsessive-compulsive disorder" or some other mental perturbation, a Christian minister would use other words: Sinners in desperate need of a Savior who have yet to experience God's grace. Twelve-step programs would charge "addiction" of whatever sort (alcohol, narcotics, food, sex, and more) and the need to come clean, from the admission of one's fundamental weaknesses and the recognition of a Higher Power to the making of amends and changes in negative behavior patterns. Thomas Moore, a monk-turned-psychoanalyst-turned-author, blames our turn-of-the-century troubles, all of them, on "loss of soul."

"When soul is neglected, it doesn't go away; it appears symptomatically in obsessions, addictions, violence, and loss of meaning," writes Moore in *Care of the Soul*. "Our temptation is to isolate these symptoms or to try to eradicate them one by one; but the root problem is that we have lost our wisdom about the soul, even our interest in it."

Unschooled in theology or psychology, unless you count church attendance, a few college courses, and a near knockdown on Fifty-second Street, I say lack of balance almost always fixates on control—our need to have control on our terms . . . *now!*

The truth is, only a tiny corner of life is ours to control. We can't control others, though we may try. We can't control the universe. We can't determine the weather. We can't push God around.

But we can decide our choices. That's powerful indeed.

Yet balanced living doesn't come naturally. We must attend to it, nurture it, grow it, as we would a flower garden. To watch life grow, to appreciate the process, is a miracle in itself, for too few of us take the time. If we did, we'd spread joy like seeds to the wind. Said philosopher Joseph Addison: "What sunshine is to flowers, smiles are to humanity. They are but trifles, to be sure, but, scattered along life's pathway, the good they do is inconceivable."

In the notorious "Top Ten" style of David Letterman, I offer a garden of balanced lifestyle choices. A tad silly, for laughter is healing. (See Number Four, below.) A tad serious, for your health of mind, mood, and body is at stake.

Most of all, I hope you find encouragement and inspiration. Power-eating, power-cising, and power-living can make a real difference in how well you think, feel, and perform. It can bring about a wonder-filled difference in you.

Just don't be in a rush.

▪ NUMBER TEN: TAKE A BREATHER ▪

Breathe in, one-two-three-four-five. Hold for five more counts and breathe out slowly. Deep, abdominal breathing is one among many relaxation techniques. Another is progressive muscle relaxation, where you tense one muscle at a time, release, and tense the next muscle and release, and so on, until after ten minutes, you're floating.

Still another is visualization. Baseball players have used it to improve batting averages, tennis players their swing, marathoners their times. Cancer patients have used it to arrest and reverse the progress of disease through enhancing the immune system. Hard to believe, but studies show that visualization influences one's physiology, including neurotransmitters, the chemical messengers that pass along vital chunks of information among your neurons.

Taking a breather is tough if you're busy. And who isn't? Surveys indicate nine out of ten adult Americans experience high stress frequently. Family doctors believe that two-thirds of all patient visits are prompted by stress-related symptoms.

The worst stress for the mind, mood, and body is the kind that drags on. The brain registers the dragging "threat" of worry, fear, or the like, which doesn't kill in a single pounce but a slow torture, and the body responds with a rush of stress hormones to gear up the body to fight or flee.

This primitive "fight or flight" response can help us jump out of the way of a speeding car, outrun a would-be attacker, or handle a sudden catastrophe. But when the release of stress hormones becomes regular, your health is jeopardized.

The antidote: relaxation.

The recurring dilemma: Who has time to relax?

I described three relaxation techniques a moment ago. Other ways to wind down include exercising, gardening, taking a warm bubble bath, reading a novel, watching a favorite flick, meditating, walking along the beach, making love—just about anything sans deadline that you really like to do.

For fun, here's an assignment: The next few days pencil "relaxation" on your calendar and learn to breathe correctly. Surprisingly, many people incorrectly perform such a basic activity. Blame it on tight clothes or sucking in the gut to appear thinner, if you must.

First, don loose-fitting clothing, lie down in a comfortable spot, and gently place your hand below your rib cage.

Next, breathe regularly and notice whether your abdomen is rising and lowering with each breath. If your chest is rising and falling instead, make a mental effort to switch your breathing to your diaphragm. Chest breathing is shallow and can cause mild to severe hyperventilation. Diaphragmatic breathing is deep and relaxing. It's the way babies and small children breathe naturally.

Finally, continue breathing, your abdomen rising and lowering, for at least ten minutes. Once you know correct breathing, you can do it anywhere, anytime, especially if you're tense. Two or three minutes of deep abdominal breathing proves relaxing.

■ Number Nine: Get Goofy ■

Why do grown men play with trains on Christmas morning?

Why do forty-somethings take to the sky in hang gliders?

Why do young lovers toss snowballs at each other?

We're loath to admit it, but we like to get silly and goof off. We have a *need* to play. Yet our culture equates play with frivolity and frivolity with a waste of precious time.

But when you teeter-totter toward too much work and too little fun, you risk losing vitality and joy. That's because play taps into an important part of you: the childlike person at your core.

Being childlike is wonderfully liberating. I think one reason people like to parent young children is they have an excuse for making silly faces, climbing on the jungle gym, and crawling through primary-colored tubes, as long as their kids are with them, that is.

We're still caught up in a belief that to be accepted as adults and be granted adult responsibilities—from credit cards and a mortgage to a coveted position as full partner in a law firm—we must act like adults.

Grown-up behavior has its place, but in embracing play, we shrug the weight of the world off our shoulders and feel light, refreshed, regenerated, invigorated, alive. Stress melts away like an ice cube in the summer sun.

Research gives a nod to goofing around too. A study of the leisure activities of some four thousand adults found that the more engaged you are in having fun, the more satisfied you are with your life.

Your assignment: Visit your neighborhood playground, hop on a swing, and go as high as you can. If you're game (and in good physical condition), jump off just like you did when you were nine years old. No playgrounds nearby? Find a tree and climb.

■ NUMBER EIGHT: SWEET DREAMS ■

Many Americans cram as many activities into twenty-four hours as possible and wear their puffy eyes and dark circles like a badge, proving just how hard-working they are. Surely someone like John Grisham would have worked late into the night on his next best-selling novel, wouldn't he? And Donna Karan on her designs, and the president on matters of state?

Me? Last night I curled up with my teddy—an overstuffed toy beaver, actually—and snoozed a full eight hours. No apologies.

Unless you're among the few who need only four to six hours of pillow time at a stretch, lack of sleep may not only turn you into a grouch but also make you physically weakened and absentminded.

Research documents the ill effects of sleepless nights: memory lapses, lack of energy, irritability, depression, anxiety, poor coordination, impaired immunity, reduced physical and mental performance, to name some. Getting ample sleep seems to have the opposite results.

In one study, for instance, researchers monitored sixty-six college-aged students before and after extending their usual sleeping time by an hour or two. The results were dramatic: The students reported better moods and greater energy after getting the extra sleep. Other research confirms that adequate sleep improves energy.

The truth is, an ongoing sleep debt drains your energy. Poor energy can cause a bad mood. Because lack of adequate sleep also affects your thinking abilities, you may have trouble making sound decisions for optimal health, like eating right and exercising.

So how much shut-eye should you get at a stretch?

The sleep experts say seven to nine hours, usually.

Though some people purposely get less sleep than they need, far more want to sleep but can't. A Gallup Poll conducted for the National Sleep Foundation found that 50 percent of Americans reported trouble sleeping some of the time and 12 percent suffered frequent insomnia.

Sleep experts offer some tips:

- Go to bed only when you're sleepy.
- Do nothing in bed but sleep. No TV viewing, no reading, nothing. The one exception: lovemaking.
- If you don't fall asleep within fifteen minutes, get up and go to another room to do something relaxing. Return to bed when you feel sleepy.
- Don't take naps during the day. Exercise instead. Research suggests that an afternoon workout improves the quality and quantity of sleep.

Your assignment: Establish a bedtime routine (a little reading, TV, or gentle stretching, don your pajamas, and brush your teeth, for example) and turn in at the same time each night. Pick the hour at which you feel moderately sleepy.

Your assignment: For several days, extend your usual sleeping time by an hour or two and log improvements in thinking, mood, energy, and other signs of wellness.

■ NUMBER SEVEN: WITH A GREAT, BIG HUG ■

". . . And a kiss from me to you. Won't you say you love me too?" These lyrics, to the tune of the kids' favorite, "This Old Man," sing-song the vitality of touch. The big, purple dinosaur got this one right: We need hugs. Lots of them, as Leo Buscaglia relates in his many books, including *Living, Loving and Learning* and *Loving Each Other*.

Buscaglia has perfected the hug. After a public speaking engagement, he walks among the people in the auditorium. A hug here, a hug there. He says, "At each lecture I encounter at least one person, attractive, often elderly, who will whisper as we embrace, 'You're the first man who has hugged me since my husband died seven years ago!' I meet men who confess to not having hugged another man, even their own sons, since they were children. 'It feels good,' they often say. One man I particularly remember, sighed, 'It's like going home again.' "

Curiously, in observing the touching habits of Americans versus Parisians, researchers discovered that in an hour's time, Parisian friends touched each other more than one hundred times, while Americans averaged three or four touches.

Human touch is essential to health. Our body chemistry changes when we are close to another person. If we fear closeness, the body pumps out stress hormones, as it does when we face danger. As we get comfortable with touch, the body responds with general feelings of well-being and relaxation. Studies have confirmed that touch deprivation often leads to despondency and a decline in functioning. Hugging can lift depression and tune up the immune system.

Hand in hand with the

TOUCH ME, HEAL ME

A friend's hug, a minister's outstretched hand, a high-five from a teammate—each communicates care, as does a special type of touch: bodywork.

Increasing in popularity, bodywork includes Swedish massage, shiatsu, reflexology, rolfing, and other types of hands-on healing. It's estimated that Americans receive 75 million massages each year. Having once been pooh-poohed as New Age mumbo jumbo, bodywork is hitting the big time.

At Columbia-Presbyterian Medical Center in New York City, patients are offered bodywork before and after surgery. It is among the more than one hundred hospitals nationwide that employ massage therapists to relieve the physical and emotional pain of patients and staffers. Bodywork is now recognized as a complementary therapy to pain management; relief from depression, anxiety, and fatigue; improved blood circulation; improved sleep; stronger immunity; and quicker recovery from injury. The Touch Research Institute at the Miami University School of Medicine says massage also has benefits for people with asthma, fibromyalgia, chronic fatigue syndrome, atherosclerosis, rheumatoid arthritis, cancer, spinal cord injuries, addictions, and other ailments.

Who should get bodywork? Everybody, say the proponents. It's hard to argue, even if massage can't deliver all of the benefits they say it can. That's because it feels fabulous.

If you decide that bodywork may help you, ask friends for a recommendation or check with a health club, a chiropractor's office, or your doctor. Check credentials too. Massage therapists must get a state license or a credential from the National Certification Board for Therapeutic Massage and Bodywork, depending on the state in which they work.

When it's time for your appointment, tell the massage therapist what you want, whether you have any particular tense or tender spots, and about medical conditions. People with high blood pressure, for instance, should get a doctor's go-ahead before a massage because it can raise blood pressure.

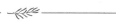

need for loving human touch is having confidants with whom we can share our deepest feelings and thoughts. Sociologists have gathered ample evidence that the healthiest and less stressed-out people have friends and family that support them. They let their guard down and reveal their true selves, warts and all, and bask in unconditional love.

The people most vulnerable to stress are those who are emotional loners. On average, they suffer more illnesses, including depression, and die at earlier ages than their well-connected peers. Sociologist James House, who analyzed data from the Tecumseh Community Health Study, calculated that social isolation was as big a risk factor for illness and death as was smoking. Scientists do not yet know the exact reason for this, but they think stress figures in.

Here's the theory in a nutshell: Being around people calms us and minimizes the fight-or-flight stress response that can bust our mind, mood, and body. In opening our hearts to one another, we can defuse the building pressure and feel loved.

Love, after all, is a universal human need.

Your assignment: Call a friend whom you haven't spent time with recently and get together. Touch on the topic of why we all need good friends and eventually make a pact, spoken or unspoken, to be there for one another. Remember to hug too.

▪ NUMBER SIX: BE STILL ▪

This is a toughie for Westerners. Our culture chants, "Go-go-go." If we're not moving, we get tagged unproductive, lazy, slothful, or worse.

I don't have to remind you that our hectic lifestyle is killing us. The medical literature on Type A's, the hard-driving, cynical, hostile perfectionists among us, is prolific and clear: Type A's are working themselves into the grave, literally.

The hard-to-swallow cure: Be still.

Being still can be as simple as relaxing in your La-Z-Boy and letting your mind flit from thought to thought without ruminating on any one. Or you can focus on your breathing or watch a candle or imagine a serene place. Or you could meditate. Easier said than done.

"Meditating makes me more edgy, not less," my friend Ann confided. When she tried to meditate, she couldn't get past the feeling that she had more important things to do—study for a test, pull weeds, scrub the toilet. Yet her boyfriend had no trouble whatsoever wiggling into the lotus position and letting his mind go blank. After thirty minutes of meditation, he felt invig-

---

5 MORE THINGS TO TRY

1. Take a catnap. Sleeping for ten to twenty minutes, but never more than forty minutes, can refresh you for several hours. Ironically, longer naps can make you feel groggy. For most people, early afternoon is the best time for a catnap because they're already a little sleepy. After your nap, count on five to twenty minutes to become fully alert.

2. Foster your creativity. When saddled with performance-oriented jobs, it's easy to squelch the playful side inherent in your personality. Find something you'd like to try—working with clay, making birdhouses, crocheting, learning the tango, making music, writing poetry—and give it a whirl. Don't concern yourself with the quality of your creative work. Instead, focus on the process.

3. Smell well. If your mom baked brownies and the scent of the chocolate perked up your after-school mood, you know a little about aromatherapy. Aromatherapy uses essential oils from plants to relax or invigorate you. Among the relaxers are lavender, chamomile, and orange blossom. Among the invigorators are spearmint, pine, or eucalyptus. Apply them to your skin or use them in bathwater.

4. Consider herbs. The herbal renaissance has given way to row after row of bottled and boxed medicinal herbs lining pharmacy shelves. Some are labeled suggestively, like "Sleepy Time." Others come right out and say what they're supposed to do. The label on St. John's Wort, among the most prescribed antidepressants in Germany, says it lifts moods. Still others just give their name: don quai, milk-thistle, chamomile, gingko, ginseng, and more. For details, check out books like *The Handbook of Medicinal Herbs* by James Duke and *The Honest Herbal* by Varro Tyler.

5. Fast. When food beckons, why choose to not eat? People have their reasons: The health-conscious may fast one to three days to detoxify their bodies, though some medical experts remain doubtful of whether fasting "detoxifies"; mourners in some cultures fast to give space to their sorrow and anger; religious people fast to observe spiritual holidays, from Judaism's Yom Kippur to Catholicism's Lent to Islam's Ramadan, or to follow the spiritual discipline of fasting and prayer. Above all, fasting is an emptying, allowing the expression of deep yearnings and spiritual growth.

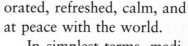

orated, refreshed, calm, and at peace with the world.

In simplest terms, meditation is a discipline in which one quiets the mind. Though it has spiritual origins, in every world religion including Christianity, Buddhism, and Hinduism, it need not be a spiritual quest. Many people use meditation to reduce stress and improve their health.

Back in 1968, Herbert Benson, M.D., studied a group of Transcendental Meditation (TM) practitioners and made some interesting discoveries: They had an increase in alpha waves (slow brain waves), a drop in blood lactate levels, and a decrease in hypometabolism (the rate of the body's oxygen consumption), all indicators of deep relaxation. Benson, who continues his research on meditation, says deep relaxation is helpful in treating any disease that stress causes or makes worse.

So how does one meditate?

Though many variations exist, a good place to start is Benson's relaxation response:

Find a quiet place and choose a time when you won't be distracted. Be sure the phone is off the hook. Sit comfortably in a chair that supports your back and head.

Then, with eyes closed, repeat a word, sound, prayer, or phrase rooted in your belief system. Focus words and phrases include the secular "one," "love," "peace," "calm," and "relax"; the Christian "let go, let God," "the Lord is my shepherd," "our Father who art in heaven"; the Jewish "shalom," "echod"; the Islamic "Insha'allah"; and the Hindu "om."

Breathe slowly and naturally and, as you do, repeat your focus word, phrase, or prayer as you exhale. When everyday thoughts come to mind, passively disregard them and return to your repetition. Continue for ten to twenty minutes.

As you finish, sit quietly for a minute or two, allowing thoughts to return. Open your eyes and sit another minute before rising. Practice the relaxation response once or twice daily.

The point is, learn to value being still and enjoy the feel-good benefits of reduced stress.

Your assignment: Follow the steps outlined above and meditate once a day for at least a week.

▪ NUMBER FIVE: LET GO ▪

Anger, guilt, shame. Bad emotions, right?

Wrong.

Please don't feel guilty if you disagree. Just hear me out. In themselves, anger, guilt, and shame are not bad. In fact, psychologists say there's no such thing as bad emotions, though there can be inappropriate expressions of them.

Rather, these emotions can teach us about who we are and what we need to do, which is often to forgive.

When we choose to hold on to anger toward another person, ourselves, or God (or all three), the person who gets maimed isn't the other. It's us. Chronic anger consumes us. It becomes our fiery sun around which we orbit.

Only in letting go of anger can we be free of it and move on.

The same is true with guilt. There are two main types: true guilt (like when we hurt someone's feelings on purpose and then feel rotten inside) and false guilt (example: Kyle and Katie blame themselves for their parents' divorce—"if only we had behaved, our family would be together"). To get beyond true guilt, amends are in order. For false guilt, we need to see it for what it is: a pretender.

And so it goes with shame. Shame is feeling so bad about oneself that you assume you have no redeeming qualities and are inherently worthless. Pond scum, slug, trash—none of these words come close to capturing the deeply painful emotion of shame.

Shame often begins in childhood. When an infant, toddler, or child hears over and over again that she's "a failure," "stupid," and "disgusting" and will "amount to nothing," she often internalizes the messages of shame and may start to believe them. The message may come through verbal, physical, or sexual abuse, or through neglect or rejection.

Overcoming shame and embracing oneself can be an arduous process. Again, at the heart of healing is forgiveness.

Forgiveness can seem impossible to extend or receive, especially when the offense is atrocious. Yet we humans, if willing, are capable of the divine.

Remember Ryan White? He was snubbed by his community, which tried to keep him out of school, though experts testified that AIDS cannot be passed through casual contact. His mother, Jeanne, forgave them. And what about Pope

---

MAKE YOUR HOME A HAVEN

Is your home what it ought to be? A place that revives and nurtures, that welcomes you back, that invites visitors to return?

A home need not be large or have skylights or expensive furniture to be a haven. But it does need love: a painting you adore above the mantel, plants on the windowsill, seashells from a vacation on the bookshelf, a child's drawing on the refrigerator, a pot of soup on the stove. To make your home a place where you can let down your hair and feel loved by family, the dog, and your own self, embrace three guidelines:

Simplify. Analyze each room, asking yourself whether each piece of furniture and every paper or knickknack stashed in a drawer really belongs. Remove what doesn't. You'll feel lighter as you unclutter.

Sense. Move around your home and sense it, literally. What do you see, smell, feel, hear, and taste? Is your personal style as exhibited in your home to your liking? Do you need a splash of your favorite color? Do you smell a potpourri of lavender? Do you feel the nubby texture of a tablecloth, hear the tinkle of a wind chime on the porch, taste the sweet of just-baked muffins?

Celebrate. A home that's a haven is a comfortable and safe place for you as well as your family and friends. Gather together as community, and celebrate a birthday, a holiday, the Sabbath, or even better, an ordinary day. When you celebrate together, you connect. You become larger, lighter, lovelier. In the words of Victoria Moran, my friend and author of *Shelter for the Spirit,* "In hosting such celebrations, a house becomes a home, and a home becomes a temple."

John Paul II? He visited his would-be assassin in jail and forgave him.

Then there are countless stories that never make the newspapers: the fifty-year-old woman who finally forgives her mother, who had robbed her of a happy childhood because she was too drunk to care; the mother of five who forgives an adulterous husband; a young father who forgives God for allowing his baby girl to die; and on and on and on.

Forgiveness is hard. But the alternative is even harder. To hold a grudge, to hang on to guilt, to embrace shame—because in some weird way, it feels good to do so—is a twenty-four-hour-a-day job. It requires intense energy. It fosters hurtful relationships. It's stressful.

I've heard forgiveness described as an eviction order, as in "I evict my anger toward so-and-so." I like that. It connotes a posture of getting up and moving forward. When you forgive (and that includes yourself) or receive forgiveness, you'll feel light, buoyant, healed.

You might not ever forget. In fact, the phrase "forgive and forget" seems outrageous. I might forgive a molester but I remember the molestation. If memories bring on anger, I can choose to forgive again. It's also unrealistic to expect instantaneous forgiveness. Often we move from "I might forgive her one day" to "I'm getting ready to forgive her" to "I will forgive this but not that" to "I forgive all."

Only then are we at peace.

Here's another assignment, a tough one: Think of a grudge you have against someone and choose to forgive or at least to consider forgiveness.

■ NUMBER FOUR: WATCH THE THREE STOOGES ■

When Norman Cousins suffered a major heart attack—and with the intimate knowledge that he had laughed, literally laughed, his way through another illness termed irreversible years before—he checked out of the hospital and began a rigorous regimen. It included a diet of very little animal fats, exercise, and a positive attitude—including hope, faith, love, will to live, cheerfulness, humor, creativity, playfulness, confidence, great expectations, and chuckles, giggles, and belly laughs.

After several months, to prove to both himself and his doctor that his heart was healing, Cousins hopped back on a treadmill in a grim little hospital room, but this time he determined to make the experience a good one. He brought a cassette.

"I asked the nurse to put on Woody Allen," Cousins shares in *The Healing Heart.* "Within a matter of seconds his offhand, mordant monologue, reinforced with audience laughter, transformed the atmosphere in the treadmill room. Dr. Shine was smiling broadly.

"Soon we would have the blood-pressure reading. I felt as though I were involved in one of those old black-and-white movies about a submarine trying to raise itself from the bottom. The captain and his lieutenants are grouped around the control panel, their eyes fixed on the depth-level indicator. . . .

" 'How are we doing?' I asked.

" 'Super,' he said.

"My heart jumped with joy. . . . All the effort and emotional investment of many months were being vindicated."

Scientists aren't exactly sure why laughing improves health of mind, mood, and body, but they've postulated some theories. Way back in the early 1900s, French physician Israel Waynbaum, the first to look at the laughter-health link, suggested that muscle contractions in the face during laughter could regulate the blood flow to the brain and, in turn, produce feelings of joy.

A decade ago, a Stanford scientist found that laughter relieves pain, much the way aerobic exercise does by boosting the endorphins. Both laughter and aerobic exercise increase heart rate and respiration. Then along came C. W. Metcalf, a self-styled humorist who charges his corporate clients up to ten thousand dollars for a seminar to teach employees how to laugh. Employers who attend are banking that a happier workplace is a healthier, less stressful, and more productive workplace.

Metcalf's first order of business: to get people over their fear of foolishness. He gets the crowd to make faces, stick out and wiggle their tongues, and let out howls. This giggle guru even convinced a group of executives to drive home after work wearing red clown noses.

Your assignment: Rent your favorite comedy, pop it in the VCR, and laugh until you're rolling in the aisles.

■ NUMBER THREE: GIVE TO GET ■

My mom was the most generous person I've ever known. Up until her death, she blessed me with her time. We'd talk for hours and never once did she seem bored of listening. At Christmas, she would go absolutely nuts showering me with presents, even in my adult years. She spoiled my husband and our daughter—her only granddaughter at the time—too.

She loved to give. More important to her than the shiny packages we gave her was watching our faces light up. Hers was boomerang generosity. You see, she grew up poor in bug-infested tenements in Chicago, and felt it her duty, once she had the means, to make sure her loved ones had *everything*.

Science bears out the goodness of giving, particularly the thing we seem to have so little of: time. One study, for instance, found that older adults who volunteered to massage preterm infants felt less anxious and depressed. They also enhanced their self-esteem and made fewer doctor visits.

When you volunteer on behalf of others, feelings of "I'm really making a difference" flood the psyche. To be effective, your contribution need not be a major sacrifice. Find something you enjoy—reading to children, manning a hotline to help new moms, gardening—then offer to help. Many communities have clearinghouses to match volunteers with groups that need their skills.

Your assignment: If you're not already experiencing the "helper's high," make a short-term commitment to volunteer doing something you enjoy. Schools, civic groups, churches, and synagogues are good places to start.

▪ NUMBER TWO: GOD, ARE YOU LISTENING? ▪

Scientists have marched into a most unlikely place to conduct their research: houses of worship.

What gives?

Simple. Mounting evidence is pointing to a surprising conclusion, surprising to secular souls, that is: Religion—and particularly prayer—is good for your health.

Some studies have looked at church attendance. They've found that people who regularly attend some kind of worship service tend to be healthier and live longer than those who never set foot inside a house of prayer. Churchgoers in general are more likely to quit smoking, cut back on alcohol, exercise more, have more friends, and stay married.

It may be argued, of course, that such changes could happen in any healthy community, not only a church, synagogue, or mosque. So let's put prayer under the microscope. As communication between the Creator and the created, it is unique to religion.

The 1988 landmark study that sparked interest in the healing power of prayer accomplished something no other prayer research had. Lead researcher Randolf Byrd used *classic scientific research methods* to evaluate the effects of intercessory prayer on nearly four hundred patients admitted to a coronary care unit.

It was a double-blind study, meaning neither participants nor the doctors knew who was being prayed for and who wasn't. The participants' names were randomly placed in the intercessory prayer group or the control group. At the start of the study, they were given scores of likely outcomes: bad, intermediate, or good.

The results amazed the medical community. The people in the intercessory prayer group were less likely to suffer congestive heart failure during recovery and had to use fewer diuretics, were less frequently intubated, and suffered fewer cases of pneumonia and cardiopulmonary arrests.

Another study examined the effect of time a hospital chaplain spent with patients. Researchers assigned about seven hundred coronary patients to one of two groups: one group received lengthy visits, averaging about an hour a day, from one of the chaplains, the other group got three-minute visits.

The results: The group with lengthy visits were discharged 1.8 to 2.1 days sooner than the others.

We all know that prayer doesn't always bring about the outcomes we may desire. A dad with cancer dies. A baby is born with Down's syndrome. A depressed person takes her life. Yet their loved ones, maybe even their doctors, prayed for healing.

So if prayer isn't always effective in healing, should doctors bother to use it as a complement to medical care?

An interesting question. I like the answer given by one researcher quoted in *Christianity Today:* "If a child comes in with leukemia, I know that 90 percent will go into remission within four weeks with vincristine and prednisone. I won't withhold these drugs because of the 10 percent who won't respond. The failure

---

PRAYER UNDER STUDY

On a prescription pad, the doctor writes out a Bible verse and hands it to the patient.

"God bless you, Doctor," the patient says.

"God bless you," the doctor replies.

This scene is repeated in a growing number of doctors' offices each day, as some members of the medical community recognize the effects of prayer on illness and disease.

The idea of praying for an ill person is nothing new, but studying prayer via classic scientific methodology is. Numerous studies are underway to determine the efficacy of prayer in healing. And as *Christianity Today* has reported, there are really one of three options: "prayer is placebo, prayer is intrinsically harmful, or prayer is intrinsically helpful. More and more evidence is supporting the last view."

So far the evidence suggests that ill people who receive prayer have better outcomes, but in general the studies to date have defined prayer generally and have not compared the advantage or disadvantage of praying to a Christian God or to Muslim's Allah or a deity of some other religion.

Though a 1996 poll for *USA Weekend* found that 79 percent of those polled believe spiritual faith can help people recover from illness, injury, and disease, and a 1997 survey by *Self* reported that 91 percent believe in miracles, few doctors take the initiative to talk to patients about spiritual matters. Honestly, there aren't many current-day precedents to guide doctors through the ethical and logistical issues of teaching patients about the curative power of prayer.

In his book *A Physician's Witness to the Power of Shared Prayer*, William Haynes, M.D., describes how he overcame his fear in opening the door to prayer. First, he simply told his patients who were being discharged from the hospital that he had prayed for them during recovery. As he gained confidence, he mentioned to his patients still in the hospital that he was praying for them nightly. Finally, he began asking patients if he could pray for them on the spot.

In a similar way, a patient could approach her doctor, mentioning her belief in God and in prayer and watching for the doctor's verbal and nonverbal response. If the doctor seems receptive, she could take a leap in faith and request prayer. Certainly, whether a doctor also believes in prayer, anyone can seek out family and friends to pray for healing.

While prayer won't necessarily bring about a cure or a good outcome, the scientific evidence suggests that some prayer may be better than no prayer.

to meet 100 percent isn't a stumbling block to a medical practitioner."

The heavenly conclusion: Some prayer seems better than no prayer, but there's no guarantee that the outcome will be the one we specifically pray for. That's the mystery.

Your assignment: Pray daily for a family member, friend, neighbor, or coworker who is sick. Let God guide your prayer: You might ask that the person be granted healing, patience, strength, and courage.

What if you don't know how to pray? Take up the challenge to learn. Ask a minister, rabbi, or other godly person for suggestions. Or simply turn to the Bible even if you aren't Christian and read what Jesus said to his disciples when they asked him to teach them to pray. He said,

This, then, is how you should pray:
"Our Father in heaven,
hallowed be your name,
Your kingdom come,
your will be done
on earth as it is in heaven.
Give us today our daily bread.
Forgive us our debts,
as we also have forgiven our
debtors.
And lead us not into temptation,
but deliver us from the evil one."
Matthew 6:9–13 (New International Version)

Many theologians say that this prayer is meant to be a model, not merely repeated formally by rote. Indeed, prayer need not be written down or have a nice rhythm. Sometimes it's simply "Help!" That's fine, because a most important aspect of prayer is that it comes from the heart.

While there are many resources from many spiritual paths, I have found these books most helpful in my own prayer life: *Too Busy Not to Pray* by Bill Hybels, *Seasons of Your Heart* by Macrina Wiederkehr, *My Utmost for His Highest* by Oswald Chambers, and *What's So Amazing About Grace?* by Philip Yancey.

▪ NUMBER ONE: HANG ON TO HOPE ▪

Remember the myth of Pandora? Zeus, who was angry with Prometheus for stealing fire from the gods, sent Pandora to earth with a box filled with many evil creatures and one good creature.

He knew the curious Pandora would open it despite his instructions not to. When she did, the creatures were unleashed. All except the good one. She replaced the lid on "hope," the great equalizer that makes life's troubles bearable.

Author C. Rick Snider defines hope as "agency," the willful determination to get what we want, and "pathways," the capability to generate the ways to get the thing we want. When you lack one or the other, hope nosedives. When you have both, it skyrockets.

My friend Dan has known hopelessness and hope. A Vietnam vet, he endured the hell of killing an elusive enemy and of watching his buddies being zipped into body bags while he lived. He coped in a narcotic fog.

He came home a war hero, but no one applauded. Most Americans hated the war and the men who fought under the red, white, and blue flag. This ex-Marine was friendless and addicted to drugs and booze. Hopelessness dragged him into a pit so deep, so dark, that he attempted suicide.

You see, he didn't know how to live anymore, so he gave up. No "pathways." No "agency." In the hospital, he went through drug rehab and hooked up with a twelve-step group. At last, he saw a way out of hell and began to hope.

He also began to regain his health: mind, mood, body, and spirit.

Research shows that hopeful people are happier and calmer. Their positive outlook on life gives them the desire and capability to set goals and solve problems. They handle stress better. They tend to get fewer illnesses, in part because they take better care of themselves, eating nutritious foods and exercising regularly.

So how do you cultivate hope?

Though genetics may come into play, becoming hopeful—or at least more so—is within your reach.

My friends Beth and Wes woke up to a nightmare: Two of their four children were diagnosed with leukemia within two weeks of each other. One received a bone marrow transplant; the other endured aggressive chemotherapy. Doctors and social workers warned them that the severe stress could pull apart their marriage.

Well aware that one or both children could die, Beth and Wes still remained hopeful. "When the doctors gave us little or no hope for Davis, who was eleven months when he was diagnosed with leukemia, our hearts and our minds still felt that hope was on our side," Beth says. "Our daughter Elisabeth Hope had the same type of bone marrow as Davis. She was a perfect match. We believe God created her that special way for a very special task—to give Davis a second chance to live."

Among their best memories, which kept them going when things got tough, was the night some fifty friends encircled their house on the coldest night of the year, holding hands with one another, singing songs of hope.

"Knowing that friends, family, and even little children cared about our boys was a tremendous source of hope and confidence," Beth adds. Both Davis and his older brother Matt are in remission.

Your assignment: Go back to the basics and evaluate how well you're taking care of your basic needs. Are you power-eating? Power-cising? Have you eliminated unnecessary "extras" that crunch your time? Are you leading a balanced life, as suggested in the Top Ten?

If you answer yes to all four, pat yourself on the back and keep up the good work. If you fall short in one or more areas, decide right now to commit yourself to accepting what you can't change and changing what you can.

You can do it. You can boost your brain power, enhance your mood, and achieve your physical peak. You can know a fuller life, a better life. You can, really.

III

Food and Recipes

Since Eve ate apples,
much depends
upon dinner

—BYRON

A Time to Celebrate

Food is yours to enjoy. Have fun in the creating and the eating and the sharing. That's right: Celebrate!

To this delicious end, read on. You'll see menus and a shopping list, and you'll get the lowdown on cutting the fat while improving flavor. And you'll learn how to power-eat in restaurants, too.

But please bury any temptation to get it all right. No one can. Just do your best, learn from your culinary flops, (you will have a few—I certainly have) and have a wonder-filled time. *Salud!*

MENUS: THINK BALANCE

When planning a menu, whether simple or gourmet, for your in-laws, a party of twenty, or a VIP—you!—remember one word: balance.

Balance brings harmony to every part of menu-planning, from the dishes you choose, to their ingredients, to the table settings, the music, and the company. So before jotting down a single word on a shopping list, ask yourself, What type of meal fits this occasion? Often you'll want a quick- and easy-to-prepare meal that's downright delicious and healthy, too. Sometimes, your deepest desire will be a sensual affair for two. Once you decide on the type of meal, consider three of the main food considerations of the balancing act: flavor, texture, and color.

Flavor. Sweet and tart, savory and fresh, spicy and mild—the tastiest meals incorporate most or all of these flavors. For instance, vegetable kebabs, bursting with the freshness of a summer garden, pairs well with savory, herbed wild rice. Corn bread tastes deliciously mild with fire-hot chili. Spiced carrot pudding combines sweet and spice in a single dish. Likewise, winter pear salad in raspberry vinaigrette marries tart and sweet, and cabbage stuffed with rice, cheese, and raisins is sweet and savory.

Texture. Did you know that when describing a food, we primarily use texture words, such as a *crisp* apple or *chewy* rice? Among the textures are crunchy, smooth, creamy, mushy, soft, and sticky. Again, go for variety and creative texture combos.

The classic green beans almandine brings together the relative softness of the beans and the crunch of toasted almonds. Soft and crunchy also come to life in a quick and popular meatless dish: a veggie burger and crusty roll topped with lettuce, tomato, and a touch of Dijon mustard, with a side of coleslaw. Chewy raisins are a welcome addition to creamy oatmeal.

Color. Picture a meal of fettuccine alfredo, mashed potatoes, and cauliflower, served with a glass of milk. What do you see? White, white, and more boring white. Now compare that meal with vegetable lasagna rollups, herbed focaccia, steamed artichokes with lemon butter, and strawberry smoothies. The latter menu paints a rainbow.

Always—and I mean *always*—make your meal visually appealing because you first feast with your eyes. But do be creative: If you want to serve an all-green dinner to celebrate St. Patrick's Day or an all-orange kids' lunch on Halloween, go for it.

Also consider the atmosphere you want to create for your meal: elegant, casual, romantic, kid-friendly, or celebratory. Select placemats, dishes, centerpieces and decorations if appropriate, and music to help set the mood. For instance, a casual dinner with good friends might call for something like this: a gingham tablecloth or placemats, earthenware dishes and chunky glasses, wildflowers in a silver vase, and jazz turned low.

I saved the best of balancing for last: nutrition. Mixing and matching the nutrients in a meal is a cinch when you stick to this simple guideline: Serve a variety of good foods (primarily grains, vegetables, fruits, legumes, nuts and seeds, and a smaller amount of animal foods) in ample portions to provide sufficient calories.

Following this guideline all but guarantees that you and the people who grace your table will eat deliciously well.

A WEEK OF MENUS

You've heard my meal-making manifesto on balance. Now *see* it. I can think of no better way than to show you a full week of menus. That means breakfast, lunch, dinner, and snacks. The meals with capitals indicate that they're among the recipes that follow. These menus show the possibilities, but in reality you probably won't follow this week's menu to a tee unless you have extra time to cook all the recipes.

SUNDAY

BREAKFAST
Buttermilk Pancakes with Fruit Toppings
Spinach-and-Feta Flan
melon balls
milk, tea, or coffee

SNACK
Cucumber Party Sandwiches
fruit juice

LUNCH*
The Best Spinach Salad
cheese wedges and crackers
tea or spritzer

SNACK
citrus fruit

DINNER
Crostini with Tomatoes, Kalamata Olives, and Basil
Seven-Vegetable Casserole
Simple Green Salad
whole-grain rolls
Not Quite Champagne

*If you eat your most substantial Sunday meal at midday, as is the tradition in some homes, flip-flop the lunch and dinner meals.

MONDAY

BREAKFAST
Banana and Granola Yogurt
fruit juice

SNACK
Carrot Bran Muffins

LUNCH
Better Gyros
kiwifruit slices

SNACK
baked potato chips

DINNER
focaccia
Capellini Pomodoro
Cinnamon Baby Carrots with Pecans
seltzer

TUESDAY

BREAKFAST
bran cereal with skim milk or soymilk
banana slices

SNACK
bagel with cream cheese

LUNCH
Creamy Broccoli Soup
crusty whole-grain bread
Cranberry-Apple Crisp
iced tea or milk

SNACK
Peanutty Oat Cookies

DINNER
Vidalia Onion Soup
Potato Pierogies and Vegetable Sauté
Chocolate Cupcakes
seltzer or tea

WEDNESDAY

BREAKFAST
Scrambled Tofu Extraordinaire
orange slices
milk, tea, or coffee

SNACK
Banana-Walnut Muffins

LUNCH
Tuscan White Bean and Herb Sandwich
baby carrots
grapes
seltzer

SNACK
Salsa Fresca with Baked Tortilla Chips
fruit juice

DINNER
Spring Rolls with Peanut Dipping Sauce
Egg Foo Yong
basmati rice
tea

THURSDAY

BREAKFAST
Raspberry-Peach Smoothie

SNACK
Nutty Apricot Muffins

LUNCH
Skinny Tostadas
brown rice
salsa
seltzer or fruit juice

SNACK
Chocolate-Banana-Almond Pudding

DINNER
Portobello Mushroom Burger
Three-Bean Salad with Honey-Mustard Dressing
pretzels
The Miracle Chocolate Chip Cookie
iced tea

FRIDAY

BREAKFAST
Blueberry Sour Cream Scones
cottage cheese
fruit
milk, tea, or coffee

SNACK
raisins
pretzels

LUNCH
Grilled Felafel Pocket
fruit juice or seltzer

SNACK
Strawberry Muffins
cheese wedges

DINNER
Spicy Sesame Noodles
Pacific Rim Coleslaw
Gingery Lemon Ice
tea

SATURDAY

BREAKFAST
Fruited French Toast
milk, tea, or coffee

SNACK
leftover muffins or cookies
fruit juice

LUNCH
PB&J Updated
baked potato chips
fruit
iced tea

SNACK
popcorn
seltzer

DINNER
Mushroom-Onion-Tomato Pizza
Frozen Banana-and-Blueberry Parfaits
seltzer

As you come across new recipes for a menu, jot down the menu and mark where to find the recipes. If so inclined, write down the menu and recipes on index cards to make a menu-and-recipe box. Having a list or recipe box will save you time in shopping and cooking.

LET'S GO SHOPPING

The delicious and healthy meals on the Power-Up Food Plan begin with the finest ingredients. To select the finest—not necessarily the most expensive!—ingredients, you'll need to become a savvy shopper. I suspect that you have down the nuts and bolts. If so, please consider this section a refresher course in shopping smart. If not, grab a cart and come along for an interesting ride.

Here are two guidelines for shopping for the finest ingredients.

Get Fresh. Unfortunately what you think is fresh—the romaine from California, the whole-wheat flour from Illinois, the grapes from South America—may not be. When foods are flown in from other states or countries, they lose valuable nutrients and flavor as they sit. More nutrients go down the drain in the many supermarkets that spray their produce with a fine mist of water to keep them looking fresh.

Your freshest bets:

- Buy produce from a farmers' market or grow some of your own food.
- Buy frozen vegetables and fruits, which go from field to a freezing facility within a few hours.
- Buy from stores with high product turnover. You're more likely to get fresh produce, flour, grains, and legumes if a store's customers snatch them up almost as fast as the clerks can stock them,
- Other ways to check for freshness before you buy: smell grains (is there a fresh or bitter odor?) and taste flour if allowed (again, is it fresh or bitter?). Bitterness suggests rancidity, which not only compromises flavor but may also create nasty free radicals in your body. Look carefully at legumes (is there cloudiness, indicating mold?). And gently handle the produce as you search for bruises, soft spots, and other early signs of rot.

Consider Organic. Ten years ago, you had to make a special trip to a natural foods store to find organic food. Now it's everywhere: Winn-Dixie, Kroger, Dominick's, Jewel, Safeway, Trader Joe's, and many other mainstream supermarkets carry foods labeled organic. But what does "organic" mean and is it really better for you?

In general, "organic" means grown without the chemical pesticides and fertilizers that most agricultural operations use to increase their yields. However, just because a product says it's "organic" doesn't mean it is. States vary widely in their rules. A handful has certification programs; nearly half lack any regulation.

When possible, buy produce certified organic. You'll all but guarantee a diet of chemical-free food. Some scientists and government groups say don't bother. They suggest that the amount of chemical residues on sprayed produce is so small it won't hurt you. Nonetheless, some studies indicate that these chemicals can slip into your fat cells and contribute to the development of diseases like cancer. Other research shows that when a breast-feeding mom eats vegetables and fruits sprayed with pesticides, it gets into her breastmilk and, in turn, her baby's tummy. Unfortunately, some of it enters his fat stores as well.

Your best bets:

- Buy foods that say "certified organic" or from farmers who you know avoid chemicals, or grow your own.
- Carefully wash foods with the highest measured pesticide levels prior to eating, or don't eat them regularly. (See "The Dirtiest Dozen, page 348.)
- Reconsider buying imported produce, which may be treated with chemicals banned for use in the United States. This may mean no strawberries in January, but you can wait until June, can't you? Ironically, some American companies peddle these banned pesticides to other countries, which spray them on their crops and sell them to American consumers—and it's all legal.

Now it's time to devise a shopping list that simplifies your grocery shopping.

THE POWER SHOPPING LIST

You can use this list as a master. Just photocopy it and, each time you plan to shop, circle the items you need. You'll save yourself time and energy—and help remind yourself of your power-eating choices.

*indicates a smart beta-carotene choice.

+indicates a smart vitamin C choice.

PRODUCE SECTION

Vegetables: artichokes, asparagus*, bamboo shoots, beans (green, lima), beets, bok choy*, broccoli*, Brussels sprouts+, cabbage (green, red), carrots*, cauliflower, celery, chard*+, collard greens*+, corn, cucumber, dandelion greens*, eggplant, kale*+, kohlrabi, leeks, lettuce, mushrooms, mustard greens*+, okra+, onion, parsnips, peas (green), peppers (sweet green+, sweet red*+), potato, pumpkin*, radishes, rhubarb, sea vegetables*+, spinach*, squash (summer, winter*), sweet potato*, tomato+, turnip, turnip greens+, water chestnuts

    Other: _____

Fruits: apple, apricots*, banana, berries (strawberries+, other varieties), cantaloupe*+, grapefruit+, grapes, guava+, honeydew melon+, kiwifruit+, lemon+, lime+, mango*+, nectarine, orange+, papaya*+, peach, pear, persimmon+, pineapple+, plantain+, plum, pomegranate, quince, sapote+, tangerine+, watermelon

    Other: _____

Fresh herbs: garlic, parsley, basil, oregano, cilantro, mint

    Other: _____

Miscellaneous: dried tomatoes, nuts (almonds, Brazil nuts, cashews, peanuts, pecans, pine nuts, walnuts), seeds (pumpkin, sesame, sunflower), tofu

    Other: _____

(Note: Nuts and seeds may also be found in the baking and snack sections.)

BREAD AND GRAIN AISLE
Whole-grain breadstuffs: bagels, bread, buns, crackers, English muffins, pita, rolls, tortillas
Brown rice
Rolled oats
Cornmeal
Other favorite whole grains: amaranth, barley, bulgur, couscous, kasha, teff
Other: _____

BAKING AISLE
Active dry yeast
Arrowroot, cornstarch or other thickener
Baking powder
Baking soda
Flours: oat, rice, rye, soy, whole-wheat, unbleached white
Peppercorns (for freshly ground black pepper)
Salt
Sweeteners: barley malt syrup, granulated sugar cane juice, honey, molasses, rice syrup, sugar
Other: _____

PACKAGED GOODS
Applesauce, unsweetened
Jam, jellies, and preserves (low-sugar or no sugar added)
Juices: apple, carrot, cranberry, orange, prune, tomato
Legumes, dried or canned: black beans, black-eyed peas, chickpeas (garbanzos), great northerns, kidney beans, lentils, pintos, split peas
Pasta
Peanut butter
Soup
Tomato paste

Tomato puree
Tomato sauce
Whole-grain cold cereals
Other: _____

CONDIMENTS, OILS, HERBS, AND SPICES
    Ketchup
    Mustard
    Olives
    Pickles
    Salsa
    Soy sauce or tamari
    Vinegars
    Other: _____
    Oils: canola, olive, peanut, safflower
    Other: _____
    Dried herbs: basil, coriander, oregano
    Spices: allspice, chili powder, cinnamon, cumin, curry, nutmeg, paprika
    Other: _____

SNACK AISLE
    Baked chips (potato, tortilla)
    Dried fruits (apricots, currants, figs, prunes, raisins)
    Popcorn kernels
    Pretzels
    Unsweetened gum
    Other: _____

DAIRY SECTION
    Butter
    Cheeses, preferably fat-reduced: cheddar, feta, Monterey Jack, mozzarella, parmesan, ricotta, romano, Swiss

Eggs
Egg substitute
Margarine, fat-reduced
Milk (buttermilk, nonfat)
Yogurt, plain
Other: _____

FROZEN FOODS
Bread dough, preferably whole grain
Pasta (ravioli, tortellini)
Vegetables (broccoli, lima beans, spinach)
Veggie burgers
Waffles, whole-grain
Other: _____

MISCELLANEOUS
Coffee
Powdered milk
Tea
Water (bottled, seltzer)
Wheat germ
Other: _____

THAI, TONIGHT?

Yes, you can power-eat at restaurants. You need to know what you want and ask for it. According to a survey by the National Restaurant Association, most restauranteurs will happily alter their cooking style on request.

But first things first: To ensure wonderful dining experiences, begin by identifying restaurants that already serve the kinds of food you want to eat. Italian and Indian eateries are smart bets. They serve many lower-fat meatless dishes. Unfortunately, most Chinese restaurants don't fit the bill. Their owners have oiled up China's ultra-healthy and delicious traditional dishes to suit American tastes. If you like Chinese food, search out an eatery willing to go very easy on the oil.

Once you've identified power-eating-friendly restaurants, make a list of them. This way you can be the first to suggest a place to eat when the subject comes up among family and friends. Don't worry about being pushy. Most people are relieved to hear another's suggestions.

Next, whether or not you end up at a power-eating-friendly establishment, learn simple tactics to get the food your mind, mood, and body needs:

- While perusing a menu, look for words like "in a fragrant broth," "topped with marinara sauce," "baked," and "grilled." Also pay attention to symbols designating a low-fat selection. Many restaurants are adding these to their menus.
- Also note words indicating dishes to avoid, like "in a cream sauce," "smothered in cheese," "triple cheese," "fried," "buttery," and "served with gravy." These dishes usually carry a heavy fat load.
- Ask questions and more questions. For instance, find out if a sauce can be omitted or replaced with a lower-fat choice, like marinara sauce or salsa, or at the very least, served on the side, so you can use as little as you choose. Another

possibility: Request extra vegetables to replace the chicken in a vegetable sauté or the beef on a kebab.

• Request that salad dressings, butter, and syrups be served on the side. This can cut down dramatically on the fat and empty calories in your meal. Use these extras sparingly.

• Be creative: You can fashion your own meal by ordering a number of appetizers and side dishes: rice and other grains (such as polenta), steamed vegetables, baked potato, vegetable soup, plain pasta, and fresh fruit. Sometimes a restaurant has items available that are not listed on the menu. Just ask.

• Beware of drinks and unhealthy breadstuffs set on your table even before you order. Alcohol and sugary drinks like soda pop are empty calories, and buttered rolls, oily breadsticks, and tortilla chips are full of fat.

• Restaurant servings are usually huge. Order a half serving if possible or split it with your dining partner. Another suggestion: Before you begin eating, set aside half of your meal in a "doggie bag" to bring home.

• Partway through your meal, stop eating and relax. It takes about twenty minutes for your brain to register that you are full. If you receive the "fullness" alert, listen.

• If you choose to eat dessert, split it with your dinner companion or wait until you get home to eat a homemade goodie.

• Splurge on occasion. As mentioned, balance is key to power-eating, so don't fall prey to the false notion of perfection. Only a power beyond yourself can rightfully claim perfection. So be human. Because you are.

All in all, when dining out, combine planning and pleasure, and you won't be disappointed.

CUT THE FAT, KEEP THE FLAVOR

A lot of people mistakenly believe that flavor must be sacrificed when you go easy on fat.

The trick to low-fat, high-flavor meals is:

- the finest ingredients
- herbs and spices
- the judicious use of wine, soy sauce, cayenne pepper sauce,
  vinegars, flavored oils, and similar ingredients in cooking
- an openness to learning new cooking methods, like sautéing
  in vegetable broth
- and time

Why time?

My personal and professional experience has taught me the value of patience and perseverance—in all things, yes, and particularly in the readjusting of one's taste buds to the fresh, unadulterated flavors of grains, vegetables, fruits, legumes, and nuts and seeds.

Adios, Fat: Say so long to too much fat by becoming fat-smart, with these chef-tested methods. Here are tips for high-flavor cooking, minus most of the fat and refined sugar:

MAIN DISHES

Cook with the freshest, most flavorful ingredients.

Use lots of fresh herbs.

Sauté in vegetable broth or red wine, or in a wee bit of oil or butter.

Use half of the cheese called for in a recipe.

Use a light sprinkling of nuts when nuts are called for in a recipe.

Replace nuts with water chestnuts (for crunch) or toasted wheat germ (for a nutty flavor) if appropriate.

Replace a whole egg with two egg whites, an equivalent amount of commercial egg substitute, or a couple tablespoons of tofu. Sometimes you can omit the egg with little effect on the recipe.

If a recipe relies heavily on high-fat ingredients (a lentil-nut loaf, for instance), find a new one.

SOUPS

Use the freshest, most flavorful ingredients.
Replace the milk or cream in creamy soups with pureed potato.

SALADS

Use the freshest, most flavorful ingredients.
Skip avocados and eggs, or use very little of them.
Dress salads very lightly in the finest olive oil and vinegar (balsamic is wonderful).
Use oil-free dressings.
Keep oil-based dressings in a dish to the side and use sparingly.

BAKED GOODS

Use flavorful fat replacers instead of half or all of the butter or margarine in a recipe. Good ones are pureed prunes (for recipes with chocolate and rich spices; you may use pureed prune baby food), pureed pears (for plain cake recipes; you may use pureed pear baby food), unsweetened apple butter (for lightly seasoned treats), and buttermilk and yogurt (use it for all the milk and half of the shortening in muffins, quick breads, and cakes).

Keep in mind that you may need to experiment a few times before your fat-reduced recipe comes out perfectly.

So Long, Sugar: Bid sugar *adieu* with these chef-tested methods.

Reduce the sugar by one-third to one-half. Consider adding tidbits of fruit like currants or minced apple for sweetness.
Replace some of the sugar with fruit juice, thawed fruit concentrate, or fruit puree. You may need to omit part of the liquid

called for in the recipe. Again, you'll need to experiment to discover what works best.

MAIN DISHES, SIDE DISHES, SALADS

With these recipes relying little on sugar, fruit juice, or thawed fruit juice concentrate in place of refined sweetener often works well.

Though vegetarian meals used to be defined by what they didn't have—meat, with all its cholesterol, saturated fats, antibiotics, and other toxins—they have become a cutting edge cuisine. Just take a look in the kitchens of the country's top chefs. They serve up dishes spiked with intensely flavored vegetables, spices, and herbs, and their patrons clamor for more. In supermarkets, foods once considered exotic, like shiitake mushrooms and jicama, are easy to find. In the media, vegetarian recipes grace the pages of every top women's magazine.

What's better, vegetarian cuisine suits power-eating to a tee. As mentioned in the previous chapters, power-eating is choosing the right foods at the right times in the right combinations. It opens the door to a brain-power boost, enhanced mood, and peak physical performance.

To this delicious end, these recipes are categorized by what they can do for you: brain boosters, energizers, stress busters, mood enhancers, PMS soothers, body builders, immunity boosters, and memory managers. To work these recipes into the Power-Up Food Plan in chapter 7, simply choose among the ones that suit your power-eating needs at any given time.

For instance, when you're on edge, grab a couple Nutty Apricot Muffins. When you need to think straight late into the night, savor Spinach and Portobello Mushroom Calzone for dinner and snack on Soy-Good Strawberry Sherbet. When you're feeling down, Chocolate Cupcakes or the Miracle Chocolate Chip Cookie can boost the endorphins, your body's "ooh-la-la" neurotransmitter, and improve your mood.

With each of the more than one hundred recipes, you'll get a nutrition breakdown. It specifies calories, carbohydrate grams, protein grams, fat grams (along with percentage of calories from fat), fiber grams, and milligrams of cholesterol and sodium for a single serving. But please resist the temptation to eat by numbers once you get the hang of the Power-Up Food Plan. As long as you power-eat—and that includes eating a variety of foods and sufficient calories—you'll get the proper amount of nutrients. So relax, and count the nutrition breakdowns as valuable information, not a dictate.

Food is yours to enjoy. Have fun in the creating and the eating and the sharing. That's right: Celebrate.

■ About the Nutrition Breakdowns ■

These aren't perfect for a simple reason: The nutrients in a given food varies according to size, length and method of storage, and other factors. With this is mind, consider the nutrition breakdowns to be close approximations, a good ballpark figure. That said, a few details:

When a recipe gives a choice of ingredients, such as butter or margarine, the first ingredient is figured in the calculations. Likewise, when there's a range of amount, such as "1 to 2 cups," the first number counts in the nutrition breakdown. Salt and black pepper are not calculated in cases of "Salt and freshly ground black pepper to taste." Neither are optional ingredients. All numbers in the breakdowns have been rounded, which may account for discrepencies between the number of calories and percentage of calories from fat. And note that the breakdowns are per serving, rather than for an entire batch.

■ Brain Boosters ■

Whenever you need mental agility—in other words, superior concentration, clear and quick thinking, enhanced creativity and insight, and an ability to reason well—brain boosters are your meal ticket. They have a healthy mix of protein and carbos and are light on fat. Among their most prominent vitamins and minerals are the B's, antioxidants, boron, iron, and zinc.

Crimini Mushroom, Tomato, and Asparagus Quiche

This healthy quiche (yes, it's possible!) combines the earthy flavor of crimini mushrooms with spring-fresh asparagus in a delicious, very low-fat crust. It's particularly rich in calcium and choline, a precursor to the brain-smart neurotransmitter acetylcholine.

CRUST:

¼ cup nonfat or part-skim
    ricotta cheese
2 tablespoons granulated sugar
1 egg white
1 tablespoon safflower or canola
    oil

½ teaspoon vanilla extract
½ cup unbleached white flour
½ cup whole-wheat flour or
    unbleached white flour
½ teaspoon baking powder
Dash salt

FILLING:

1 tablespoon butter
2 tablespoons Basic Vegetable
    Stock (page 247)
1½ cups diced crimini
    mushrooms
½ onion, diced
1 cup evaporated skim milk
½ cup egg substitute or 2 eggs
⅓ cup reduced-fat shredded
    Swiss cheese

¼ teaspoon ground nutmeg
Freshly ground black pepper to
    taste
⅔ cup freshly grated Parmesan
    cheese
2 plum tomatoes, sliced thinly
6 asparagus spears, lightly
    steamed

SERVES 6

CRUST: In a large bowl, combine the ricotta, sugar, egg white, oil, and vanilla. Stir in the flours, baking powder, and salt until just combined.

Preheat the oven to 350 degrees. On a lightly floured surface, roll out the dough to make a circle one inch larger than the quiche dish or pie pan. Bake 7 minutes. Set aside.

FILLING: In a skillet, heat the butter and vegetable stock over medium heat. Add the mushrooms and onion, and sauté until the onion is transparent, about 10 minutes. Meanwhile, in a medium bowl, combine the milk, egg substitute or eggs, cheese, nutmeg, and black pepper. Stir in the mushroom mixture. Set aside.

Sprinkle ⅓ cup Parmesan on the bottom of the crust. Place half of the tomato slices on top. Pour in the mushroom-egg mixture. Arrange the asparagus spears in a spoke-wheel design. Dip both sides of the remaining tomato slices in the remaining Parmesan. Place the tomato slices between the spokes. Bake until set, about 1 hour. Serve warm.

> PER SERVING: 307 calories; 14g protein; 45g carbohydrates; 9g fat (26 percent calories from fat); 3g fiber; 21mg cholesterol; 638mg sodium.

Basic Vegetable Stock

A rich homemade stock can turn a good recipe into pure heaven. The vegetables should be well washed and ripe but not rotting, and the water pure with no odor of chlorine or anything else.

Store-bought powdered vegetable broth mix available in natural food stores may stand in for homemade if you have neither stock on hand nor the time to simmer up a pot or if it plays a very minor role in the recipe. For instance, reach for a jar of powdered vegetable broth mix if you're substituting a tablespoon or two of stock for fat in a sauté.

The easiest way to stock up on stock is to freeze it in small portions—one-half to one cup—so you can add it for a flavor kick as needed. Employ an ice cube tray for tinier amounts. Just pour in the stock, freeze, then transfer to a large Ziploc bag.

One more thought, if you do not have these vegetables on hand, use others except strong-tasting ones like broccoli and beets.

1 tablespoon virgin olive oil
3 onions, cut into eighths
1 tablespoon minced fresh garlic
4 celery stalks, including leaves,
    chopped
2 leeks, including greens,
    chopped
2 turnips, chopped
4 potatoes, chopped
3 carrots, chopped
12 cups cold water

2 bay leaves
2 tablespoons minced fresh
    thyme leaves (or 2 teaspoons
    dried)
2 tablespoons chopped fresh
    parsley leaves
6 whole cloves
Other fresh or dried herbs as
    desired
Salt and freshly ground black
    pepper to taste

MAKES 12 CUPS

In a large soup pot, heat the oil over medium heat. Add the vegetables and cook about 15 minutes, stirring occasionally. Pour in the water, add the seasonings, and bring to a simmer. Cover and cook for at least 1 hour. (The longer it simmers, the more robust the flavor.) Set a colander over a large bowl. Pour in the stock. With a wooden spoon, push against the vegetables to extract the juices. Discard the vegetables, bay leaves, and cloves.

Use right away or store it in an airtight container in the refrigerator for up to three days or in the freezer for up to six months.

Spinach-and-Feta Flan

With distinctive Greek flavor, this flan is a cinch to make and boasts a hefty dose of antioxidants, iron, and calcium.

6 cups spinach, trimmed and
    chopped
1 cup nonfat or part-skim ricotta
    cheese
1 cup low-fat cottage cheese

2 eggs, lightly beaten, or ½ cup
    egg substitute
Dash ground nutmeg
⅓ cup crumbled feta cheese
Salt and freshly ground black
    pepper to taste

SERVES 4

Preheat the oven to 350 degrees. Steam the spinach until just wilted and set aside to cool slightly. In a medium bowl, mix together the cheeses, eggs or egg substitute, and nutmeg. Add the spinach and thoroughly combine. Pour into a nonstick 8- or 9-inch pie pan. Sprinkle the feta on top.

Bake until set, about 40 minutes. Season with the salt and pepper. Serve warm.

PER SERVING: 202 calories; 26g protein; 9g carbohydrates; 7g fat (31 percent calories from fat); 2g fiber; 133mg cholesterol; 636mg sodium.

Scrambled Tofu Extraordinaire

With the addition of vegetables and herbs, ordinary scrambled tofu gets a flavor- and vitamin-boost. It is rich in beta-carotene and vitamin C.

¾ cup broccoli florets
½ onion, chopped
1 teaspoon minced fresh garlic
½ red bell pepper, cored and diced
2 tablespoons Basic Vegetable Stock (page 247)
One 10½-ounce package reduced-fat firm tofu, drained and crumbled

2 tablespoons fresh tarragon (or 2 teaspoons dried)
¼ teaspoon celery seed
½ to 1 teaspoon turmeric
Dash white pepper
2 teaspoons butter or reduced-fat margarine

SERVES 4

Lightly steam the broccoli until barely tender, about 3 minutes. Set aside. In a saucepan, cook the onion, garlic, and red bell pepper in the vegetable stock until the stock is almost evaporated, about 5 minutes. In a bowl, thoroughly combine the tofu and spices. Stir in the vegetables.

Heat the butter or margarine over medium heat in a large skillet. Add the tofu mixture. Sauté until heated through, stirring gently with a spatula, about 5 minutes.

Smart Note: Tofu is a nutritionist's dream. It's packed with health-promoting phytochemicals that may protect against some diseases. But tofu may take some getting used to. If you're among the uninitiated, try it first in dishes where it plays a supporting role, such as Broccoli Dip with Marinated Sun-Dried Tomatoes and Brazil Nuts (page 264).

> PER SERVING: 79 calories; 9g protein; 5g carbohydrates; 3g fat (34 percent calories from fat); 2g fiber; 6mg cholesterol; 133mg sodium.

Golden Potato Chowder

Cheese lovers unite: This soup has only 10 grams of fat per big bowl.

3 cups peeled and cubed red potatoes
½ cup sliced celery
½ cup grated carrots
¼ cup chopped onion
1½ cups Basic Vegetable Stock (page 247)
½ teaspoon salt (optional)
Freshly ground black pepper to taste

One 12-ounce can evaporated skim milk
2 tablespoons whole-wheat flour or unbleached white flour
1 cup shredded reduced-fat cheddar cheese
1 tablespoon chopped fresh parsley

SERVES 4

In a saucepan, combine the potatoes, celery, carrots, onion, vegetable stock, salt if desired, and black pepper. Bring to a boil, cover, and simmer for 20 minutes. Add the milk to the flour a little bit at a time while stirring. Pour the milk mixture into the chowder. Let simmer until thickened, about 10 minutes. Remove from the heat. Stir in the cheese until melted. Pour the chowder into four bowls. Sprinkle with the parsley.

PER SERVING: 351 calories; 28g protein; 39g carbohydrates; 10g fat (26 percent calories from fat); 3g fiber; 44mg cholesterol; 581mg sodium.

Vegetable Cassoulet

Cassoulet is a renowned dish from southern France. This hearty version plays up legumes and not goose or duck or sausage.

1 cup dried navy beans, soaked
   overnight in water to cover
3 cups water
1 onion, thickly sliced

1 or 2 cloves garlic, halved
Salt and freshly ground black
   pepper to taste

1 cup thickly sliced white button
   mushrooms
2 carrots, sliced
1 stalk celery, sliced
1 cup tomato puree
3 tablespoons chopped fresh
   oregano (or 1 teaspoon dried)
½ cup shredded mozzarella cheese

⅓ cup low-fat cottage cheese
⅓ cup part-skim ricotta cheese
One 10-ounce package frozen
   chopped spinach, thawed
¼ cup shredded fresh Parmesan
   cheese
⅓ cup dry bread crumbs,
   preferably whole wheat

SERVES 6

In a large saucepan, combine the beans (first draining off the overnight soaking water), water, onion, and garlic. Bring to a boil over medium-high heat, reduce to medium-low, cover, and simmer until the beans are just tender, about 40 minutes. Discard the garlic. Season with the salt and pepper. Set aside. In a medium bowl, combine the mushrooms, carrots, celery, tomato puree, oregano, and mozzarella. Combine the cottage cheese and ricotta cheese in another bowl. Set aside.

Heat the oven to 375 degrees. Spread half of the bean mixture in a lightly oiled 2-quart casserole. Cover with half of the spinach, half of the cheese mixture, and half of the vegetable mixture. Repeat the layers. Sprinkle the Parmesan and bread crumbs on top. Bake until bubbly and the cheese melts, about 45 minutes.

> PER SERVING: 283 calories; 20g protein; 42g carbohydrates; 5g fat (16 percent calories from fat); 9g fiber; 15mg cholesterol; 565mg sodium.

Better Gyros

American-style gyros are made with lamb and lots of fatty add-ons. Here's a delicious vegetable-and-chickpea version.

2 tablespoons fresh lemon juice
1 to 2 tablespoons minced fresh garlic
One 15-ounce can chickpeas
2 tablespoons red wine or Basic Vegetable Stock (page 247)
2 cups thinly sliced onions
1½ cups sliced crimini mushrooms
1 red bell pepper, cored and sliced into thin strips

1 yellow bell pepper, cored and sliced into thin strips
Eight 8-inch pita rounds
⅓ cup chopped Kalamata olives
1 cup chopped plum tomatoes
½ cup crumbled feta cheese
¼ cup chopped fresh basil
Freshly ground black pepper to taste

MAKES 8

Place the lemon juice and garlic in a blender or a bowl. Drain the chickpeas, reserving 2 tablespoons of liquid. Add the chickpeas and reserved liquid to the blender or bowl. Blend until smooth. (Or use a fork to mash the juice, garlic, and chickpeas in the bowl, mixing until smooth.) Set aside.

Heat the red wine or stock over medium heat, and sauté the

onions, mushrooms, and bell peppers until tender, about 8 minutes, adding more wine or stock as needed.

Wrap the pitas in paper towels and heat in a microwave about 45 seconds. (If you'd rather warm the pitas in your oven, simply stack them and cover them with a damp dish towel and heat for 10 minutes at 300 degrees.) Spread 2 tablespoons of the bean mixture over each pita round, and top with the vegetable mixture, olives, tomatoes, cheese, basil, and black pepper. Fold in half and secure with a toothpick. Serve warm.

PER SERVING: 290 calories; 12g protein; 50g carbohydrates; 6g fat (19 percent calories from fat); 6g fiber; 13mg cholesterol; 489mg sodium.

Spinach and Portobello Mushroom Calzone

This recipe got raves from the men and women in one of my cooking classes, few of whom were vegetarian. It's surprisingly meaty and deeply flavorful. Incidentally, using store-bought frozen bread dough as the wrap makes the preparation surprisingly simple. Here's the first of three uniquely flavored calzone recipes.

1 pound frozen bread dough, thawed

2 tablespoons red wine or Basic Vegetable Stock (page 247)

1 onion, diced

2 teaspoons minced fresh garlic

1 portobello mushroom, chopped

One 10-ounce package frozen chopped spinach, thawed

2 cups part-skim ricotta cheese

¼ cup shredded part-skim mozzarella cheese

¼ cup grated fresh Parmesan cheese

Freshly ground black pepper to taste

2 cups warmed Quick Marinara Sauce (page 255), or your favorite store-bought pasta sauce

MAKES 4

Divide the bread dough into four equal balls. Lightly flour your work surface. Roll out a ball into an eight-inch circle. Repeat with the remaining dough, cover with waxed paper, and set aside.

> **HIGH-CHOLINE FOODS**
>
> Wheat germ
> Soybeans
> Peanuts
> Peanut butter
> Whole-wheat flour
> Egg yolk
> Pecans

In a large saucepan, heat the wine or stock over medium heat and simmer the onion, garlic, and mushroom until the liquid evaporates, about 10 minutes. Stir in the spinach, cheeses, and black pepper. Set aside.

Preheat the oven to 400 degrees. Spoon one-fourth of the mushroom-spinach mixture onto half of a dough circle, leaving a one-half-inch edge. Fold the dough over the filling, and seal by crimping the edges with a fork. Place the calzone on a baking sheet lightly coated with cooking spray. Repeat with the remaining mushroom-spinach mixture and dough circles.

Bake until golden, about 20 minutes. Set each calzone on a plate. Ladle the sauce over the calzones.

PER SERVING: 502 calories; 38g protein; 76g carbohydrates; 6g fat (11 percent calories from fat); 7g fiber; 14mg cholesterol; 735mg sodium.

Quick Marinara Sauce

You can personalize this sauce: Stir in fresh herbs from your garden, add chopped olives, toss in capers, sauté some exotic mushrooms along with the vegetables, whatever suits your culinary fancy.

2 teaspoons virgin olive oil	1 teaspoon dried oregano
1 small onion, diced	1 teaspoon dried basil
1 teaspoon minced fresh garlic	Dash cayenne pepper
⅓ cup minced green bell pepper	½ cup water
1 carrot, shredded	Salt and freshly ground black
One 8-ounce can tomato sauce	pepper to taste
One 6-ounce can tomato paste	

MAKES 2 CUPS; 4 SERVINGS

In a medium saucepan, heat the olive oil over medium-high heat. Sauté the onion, garlic, green bell pepper, and carrot until the onion is transparent, about 5 minutes. Reduce the heat to medium. Add the remaining ingredients and cook 5 to 10 minutes more. Serve warm.

PER SERVING: 93 calories; 3g protein; 17g carbohydrates; 3g fat (29 percent calories from fat); 0mg cholesterol; 635mg sodium.

Sun-Dried Tomato and Olive Calzone

The sweetness of the sun-dried tomatoes plays off the olives wonderfully. This dish boasts calcium, vitamin C, and phytochemicals.

1 pound frozen bread dough,
  thawed
2 tablespoons Basic Vegetable
  Stock (page 247)
2 scallions (white and green
  parts), sliced
2 teaspoons minced fresh garlic
¼ cup sun-dried tomatoes
  packed in oil, drained and
  blotted dry
¼ cup pitted black olives,
  chopped
2 cups nonfat or part-skim
  ricotta cheese

½ cup shredded reduced-fat
  Monterey Jack cheese
¼ cup shredded fresh Parmesan
  cheese
1 cup minced fresh herbs, such as
  parsley, basil, oregano
Freshly ground black pepper to
  taste
2 cups warmed Quick Marinara
  Sauce (page 255) or your
  favorite store-bought pasta
  sauce

MAKES 4

Divide the bread dough into four equal balls. Lightly flour your work surface. Roll out a ball into an eight-inch circle. Repeat with the remaining dough, cover with waxed paper, and set aside.

In a large saucepan, heat the wine or stock over medium heat and simmer the scallions and garlic until the liquid evaporates, about 5 minutes. Stir in the tomatoes, olives, cheeses, herbs, and pepper. Set aside.

HIGH–BETA-CAROTENE FOODS

Pumpkin
Sweet potato
Carrot
Mango
Spinach
Papaya
Cantaloupe
Kale
Dried apricots
Collards
Tomato
Asparagus

Preheat the oven to 400 degrees. Spoon one-fourth of the sun-dried tomato-olive mixture onto half of a dough circle, leaving a one-half-inch edge. Fold the dough over the filling, and seal by crimping the edges with a fork. Place the calzone on a baking sheet lightly coated with cooking spray. Repeat with the remaining sun-dried tomato-olive mixture and dough circles.

Bake until golden, about 20 minutes. Set each calzone on a plate. Ladle the sauce over the calzones.

PER SERVING: 550 calories; 41g protein; 71g carbohydrates; 11g fat (18 percent calories from fat); 28mg cholesterol; 835mg sodium.

Broccoli and Onion Calzone

I like the combination of broccoli and perfectly sautéed onions in many dishes, especially pizza and calzone. There are loaded with beta-carotene and phytochemicals.

1 pound frozen bread dough, thawed
¼ cup dry white wine or Basic Vegetable Stock (page 247)
2 onions, sliced
2 teaspoons minced fresh garlic
One 10-ounce package frozen chopped broccoli, thawed
2 cups nonfat or part-skim ricotta cheese

½ cup shredded part-skim mozzarella cheese
¼ cup shredded fresh Parmesan cheese
½ cup chopped fresh parsley
Freshly ground black pepper to taste
2 cups warmed Quick Marinara Sauce (page 255) or your favorite store-bought pasta sauce

MAKES 4

Divide the bread dough into four equal balls. Lightly flour your work surface. Roll out a ball into an eight-inch circle. Repeat with the remaining dough, cover with waxed paper, and set aside.

In a large saucepan, heat the wine or stock over medium heat, and simmer the onions and garlic until the onion is softened, adding more stock as necessary, about 10 minutes. Stir in the broccoli, cheeses, parsley, and pepper. Set aside.

Preheat the oven to 400 degrees. Spoon one-fourth of the broccoli-onion mixture onto half of a dough circle, leaving a one-half-inch edge. Fold the dough over the filling, and seal by crimping the edges with a fork. Place the calzone on a baking sheet lightly coated with cooking spray. Repeat with the remaining broccoli-onion mixture and the remaining dough circles.

Bake until golden, about 20 minutes. Set each calzone on a plate. Ladle the sauce over the calzone.

PER SERVING: 543 calories; 37g protein; 83g carbohydrates; 7g fat (12 percent calories from fat); 8g fiber; 58mg cholesterol; 873mg sodium.

Egg Foo Yong

Take-out egg foo yong is oil-heavy and, well, not nearly as tasty as these vegetable-studded egg pancakes. It's rich in antioxidants and choline, a precursor to the brain-smart neurotransmitter acetylcholine.

GRAVY:

2 teaspoons canola or safflower oil
1 to 2 cups fresh shiitake mushrooms or white button mushrooms
1 teaspoon cornstarch
1½ cups Basic Vegetable Stock (page 247)
1 teaspoon minced fresh garlic
1 teaspoon peeled and grated gingerroot
1 tablespoon low-sodium soy sauce or tamari, or to taste
1 teaspoon honey

PATTIES:

3 eggs, beaten
1 cup mashed reduced-fat firm
  silken tofu
¼ cup sherry or Basic Vegetable
  Stock (page 247)
1 stalk celery, cut lengthwise and
  sliced thinly on the diagonal
½ cup chopped fresh shiitake
  mushrooms
½ cup sliced white button
  mushrooms

4 scallions (green and white
  parts), chopped
2 cups fresh bean sprouts
¼ cup diced water chestnuts
1 teaspoon peeled and minced
  gingerroot
1 to 2 teaspoons peanut oil or
  sesame oil
Low-sodium soy sauce or tamari
  to taste

MAKES 9; SERVES 3

GRAVY: In a medium skillet, heat the oil over medium-high heat. Sauté the mushrooms for 10 minutes. In a small bowl, combine the cornstarch with a few tablespoons of the stock. Bring the remaining gravy ingredients to a gentle boil in a small saucepan, add the diluted cornstarch, reduce the heat to medium-low, and cook until thickened, about 5 minutes. Set aside.

PATTIES: In a blender or food processor, whirl the eggs and mashed tofu until very smooth. The batter should be slightly thinner than pancake batter. Set aside.

In a wok or large saucepan, combine the sherry or stock, celery, mushrooms, and scallions and cook, stirring occasionally, until the liquid is almost evaporated, about 5 minutes. Stir in the

HIGH-THIAMINE FOODS

Rice bran
Whole-wheat flour
Wheat germ
Black beans
Navy beans
Split peas
Black-eyed peas
Lentils
Oat bran
Lima beans
Brazil nuts
Kidney beans
Soybeans
Pine nuts
Green peas
Chickpeas
Brown rice
Tahini

remaining ingredients except the oil and soy sauce. Sauté until
tender-crisp, about 3 minutes.

Add the vegetables to the egg mixture and combine them. Heat
the oil in a skillet over medium heat, swirling the skillet to coat the
bottom. Drop in the batter by large spoonfuls, forming small
pancake-sized rounds. Cook until browned on the bottom, about 3
minutes. Turn over and cook the other side until browned, another
3 minutes. Repeat with the remaining batter. Season with the soy
sauce. Serve at once with the gravy.

PER SERVING: 274 calories; 18g protein; 23g carbohydrates; 11g fat
(36 percent calories from fat); 212mg cholesterol; 370mg sodium.

▪ ENERGIZERS ▪

When you're wondering where your get-up-and-go got up and
went, choose an energizer. Its carbo-protein mix keeps the amino
acid tryptophan at bay so your brain can get ample dopamine
and norepinephrine, along with the B vitamins, vitamin C, and
the minerals potassium, magnesium, iron, and selenium. Steer
clear of refined sugar, which can monkey with your blood sugar
levels. Caffeine in moderation is an acceptable pick-me-up.

Sunny Pecan Granola

Enjoy this makeover of the original high-fat breakfast cereal with
skim milk or fortified soymilk.

3 cups rolled oats
¼ cup sunflower seeds
¼ cup chopped pecans
¼ cup toasted wheat germ
12 dried apricot halves, diced
⅓ cup honey

2 tablespoons molasses,
  preferably blackstrap
¼ cup calcium-fortified orange
  juice
Other chopped dried fruit, such
  as apples and bananas
  (optional)

MAKES 8 ONE-HALF-CUP SERVINGS

Preheat the oven to 325 degrees. Place the oats in a baking pan in an even layer no more than 1-inch deep. Bake 5 to 10 minutes, stirring occasionally, until warmed through and crisp to the bite.

Combine with the sunflower seeds, pecans, and wheat germ. In a small saucepan, heat the apricots, honey, molasses, orange juice, and other dried fruit, if using, until warm, about 3 minutes. Add to the oat mixture and combine thoroughly.

Spread in a baking pan in a one-inch-thick layer. Bake, stirring occasionally, until golden brown, about 20 minutes. Let cool. Store in an airtight container.

PER SERVING: 266 calories; 8g protein; 45g carbohydrates; 7g fat (24 percent calories from fat); 6g fiber; 0mg cholesterol; 7mg sodium.

Banana-and-Granola Yogurt

My friend Jennifer, a schoolteacher who has little time for a sit-down breakfast, gave me the idea for this protein-rich tote-able morning meal or snack.

1 cup store-bought low-fat granola or Sunny Pecan Granola (page 260)
1 banana, cut lengthwise in quarters and sliced thickly

½ cup plain or vanilla nonfat yogurt

SERVES 2

In an airtight container with a cover, gently mix together all the ingredients. Serve at once or chill. If you're eating it away from home, don't forget a spoon.

PER SERVING: 294 calories; 9g protein; 61g carbohydrates; 3g fat (9 percent calories from fat); 4g fiber; 1mg cholesterol; 162mg sodium.

Fruited French Toast

What we call French toast is a dessert in France by the name *pain perdu,* or lost bread. It's made of stale (i.e., lost) bread soaked in rich milk and lots of eggs, then fried. This update nixes most of the fat and retains an alluring texture and flavor.

FRUIT:

1 cup fruit-flavored nonfat yogurt (blended, not fruit-on-the-bottom)
2 tablespoons fruit preserves

TOAST:

2 eggs
2 egg whites
¼ cup reduced-fat soymilk or skim milk
½ teaspoon vanilla extract
8 slices of Italian bread, diagonally cut 1 inch thick

SERVES 4

FRUIT: Line a sieve with several layers of cheesecloth. Pour the yogurt into the sieve and place it over a bowl in the refrigerator to drain overnight. Transfer the strained yogurt to a small bowl and stir in the fruit preserves. Set aside.

TOAST: In a shallow bowl, beat together the eggs and egg whites with a whisk or fork until foamy. Add the soymilk or skim milk, and vanilla. Preheat the oven to 200 degrees. Lightly oil a large nonstick skillet and place over medium heat. Dip four bread slices into the egg mixture, turning to coat. Arrange on the skillet and cook until golden, turning once, about 2 or 3 minutes per side. Place them in a single layer on an oven-proof plate and keep them warm in the oven as you cook the remaining toasts.

HIGH-RIBOFLAVIN FOODS

Soybeans
Yogurt
Cottage cheese
Almonds
Whole or skim milk
Ricotta cheese
Wheat germ
Cheese

Divide the French toast among the plates and spread some fruited yogurt on each. Serve at once.

Smart Note: Soymilk bursts with phytochemicals and other goodies that scientists continue to discover more about. And in baked goods it's indistinguishable from dairy milk.

> PER SERVING: 271 calories; 12g protein; 44g carbohydrates; 5g fat (17 percent calories from fat); 2g fiber; 107mg cholesterol; 417mg sodium.

Zucchini-Stuffed Mushrooms

This quick appetizer is an elegant pick-me-up. The pine nuts and low-fat cheeses give a protein boost while the zucchini and mushrooms supply fiber and vitamins.

1 tablespoon Basic Vegetable Stock (page 247) or dry white wine

12 large white mushrooms, stems removed and chopped

1 teaspoon minced fresh garlic

1 scallion (green and white parts), chopped

2 medium zucchini, shredded and set in a colander to drain

Extra Basic Vegetable Stock as needed

½ cup nonfat or part-skim ricotta cheese, or soft silken tofu

¼ cup freshly grated Parmesan cheese

⅓ cup dry bread crumbs, preferably whole wheat

¼ teaspoon dried oregano

Freshly ground black pepper to taste

2 tablespoons lightly toasted pine nuts for garnish (see tip, below)

SERVES 4

In a medium skillet, heat the vegetable stock or wine over medium heat and sauté the mushroom stems, garlic, and scallion until softened, about 5 minutes. Squeeze the zucchini to remove excess liquid, add to the skillet, and sauté another 5 minutes, adding vegetable stock as needed. Remove from the heat.

Preheat the oven to 350 degrees. In a small bowl, whisk together the ricotta or tofu, Parmesan, bread crumbs, oregano, and pepper. Add to the skillet and combine. Stuff the zucchini mixture into the hollows of the mushrooms. Place them on a lightly oiled baking sheet, garnish with the pine nuts, and bake 15 minutes. Serve warm.

A Tip: To toast nuts and seeds, heat a small skillet over medium-high heat, add the pine nuts, and gently shake the pan until the nuts are lightly browned, about 2 or 3 minutes.

> PER SERVING: 134 calories; 11g protein; 13g carbohydrates; 5g fat (33 percent calories from fat); 2g fiber; 5mg cholesterol; 216mg sodium.

Broccoli Dip with Marinated Sun-Dried Tomatoes and Brazil Nuts

You can't taste the tofu in this dip. Serve it with your favorite whole-grain crackers and delight in knowing you're getting the amazing phytochemicals in soybeans.

5 ounces reduced-fat firm or soft silken tofu

4 ounces nonfat or reduced-fat cream cheese

1 to 2 tablespoons minced fresh garlic

1 teaspoon vegetarian Worcestershire sauce (see tip, opposite page)

One 10-ounce package frozen chopped broccoli, lightly steamed and drained

2 to 4 tablespoons sun-dried tomatoes packed in oil, drained and blotted dry

1 tablespoon chopped and toasted Brazil nuts

MAKES 2 CUPS; SERVES 16

In a medium bowl, whisk together the tofu, cream cheese, garlic, and Worcestershire sauce. Add the broccoli and sun-dried tomatoes. Chill at least 1 hour. Garnish with the nuts before serving.

A Tip: Vegetarian Worcestershire sauce contains no anchovies. Look for it in natural food stores.

PER SERVING: 25 calories; 3g protein; 2g carbohydrates; 1g fat (30 percent calories from fat); 1g fiber; 1mg cholesterol; 50mg sodium.

Garlicky Pita Toasts

These protein-enhanced toasts are a delicious appetizer or accompaniment to soups.

4 pita rounds
1 egg white
1 tablespoons virgin olive oil
¼ cup chopped fresh parsley

¼ cup freshly grated Parmesan cheese
2 teaspoons minced fresh garlic

MAKES 32; SERVES 8

Preheat the oven to 300 degrees. Cut each pita round into quarters. Then pull apart the bread to make a total of thirty-two pieces. Place in a single layer on cookie sheets.

In a small bowl, beat the egg white until frothy. Stir in the remaining ingredients. Spread over the rough side of the pita. Bake until the cheese melts and the edges are toasted, about 10 minutes. Let cool.

Smart Note: To make fewer toasts, simply cut the ingredients in half and proceed as directed.

> PER SERVING: 115 calories; 5g protein; 18g carbohydrates; 3g fat (23 percent calories from fat); 2g fiber; 2mg cholesterol; 224mg sodium.

Spanakopita Triangles

A fabulous fat-laden and time-consuming Greek dish gets slimmed down and simplified in this version. It's rich in iron, calcium, choline, and beta-carotene. Serve it as an appetizer, snack, or light lunch.

¼ cup dry white wine or sherry
1 onion, chopped
3 cups fresh spinach leaves, trimmed
2 tablespoons salt
1 egg
¼ cup low-fat cottage cheese

½ cup crumbled feta cheese
Freshly ground black pepper to taste
8 sheets phyllo (see tip, below)
1 tablespoon melted butter
Butter-flavored cooking spray

MAKES 12; SERVES 4

In a skillet, heat the wine or sherry over medium heat and sauté the onion until softened, about 5 minutes. Chop the spinach. Place it in a bowl and sprinkle the salt all over. Wring it with your hands to wilt it. Place it in a sieve and rinse it well. Squeeze dry. In a bowl, combine the onion, spinach, egg, cheeses, and pepper.

HIGH–VITAMIN B$_6$ FOODS

Avocados
Bananas
Wheat bran
Rice bran
Carrots
Filberts
Lentils
Brown rice
Soybeans
Wheat germ
Whole-grain flour

Preheat the oven to 350 degrees. Lightly oil a baking sheet. On a clean surface, stack the sheets of phyllo with a short end toward you. Cut lengthwise with kitchen scissors into thirds, and stack the strips in one pile. Very lightly brush the two top strips with butter. Place about a tablespoon of the filling at the end closest to you. Fold a corner of the two strips over the filling diagonally to make a triangle. Continue folding, as if it were a flag. Place the triangle on the prepared baking sheet. Lightly coat the top with the cooking spray.

Repeat this same procedure with the remaining strips and filling. Bake until golden, about 12 minutes.

A Tip: Phyllo (also spelled *filo*) dries quickly, so be sure to cover the reserved pieces with a slightly damp clean cloth.

> PER SERVING: 276 calories; 12g protein; 34g carbohydrates; 10g fat (33 percent calories from fat); 4g fiber; 35mg cholesterol; 1,156mg sodium.

Skinny Tostadas

The cheddar cheese and black beans give this light lunch or dinner a one-two protein punch.

Eight 10-inch tortillas, preferably whole wheat
½ cup nonfat sour cream
1 teaspoon chili powder
½ teaspoon ground cumin
1 teaspoon minced fresh garlic
One 4-ounce can green chilies

1 cup shredded reduced-fat Monterey Jack cheese
1 cup cooked black beans
3 fresh plum tomatoes, diced
¼ cup chopped scallions (green and white parts)

SERVES 4

Preheat the oven to 350 degrees. Wrap the tortillas in a slightly damp dish towel and warm in the oven for a few minutes. Meanwhile, in a small bowl, mix together the sour cream, chili powder, cumin, garlic, and chilies. Place four tortillas on a baking sheet. Spread the sour cream mixture on top. Sprinkle the cheese, beans, tomatoes, and scallions on top. Place the remaining four tortillas on top to make sandwiches. Bake until the cheese melts, about 3 to 5 minutes. Serve warm.

> PER SERVING: 347 calories; 20g protein; 50g carbohydrates; 10g fat (26 percent calories from fat); 6g fiber; 23mg cholesterol; 903mg sodium.

Quick Black Bean Burritos

Need a speedy dinner? This dish pairs legumes and cheese with healthy carbos—and it's ready in just twenty minutes.

SAUCE:

½ onion, chopped
1 teaspoon minced fresh garlic
½ teaspoon ground cumin
One 14½-ounce can diced
    tomatoes

1 to 2 tablespoons minced green
    chilies, fresh or canned, seeded
¼ cup chopped fresh cilantro

BURRITOS:

Eight 10-inch flour tortillas,
    preferably whole wheat
One 15-ounce can black beans,
    drained and rinsed
½ red onion, diced
¾ cup cooked brown rice

¾ cup shredded reduced-fat
    sharp cheddar cheese
½ cup nonfat sour cream
½ avocado, diced (optional)
2 tablespoons fresh cilantro
    leaves for garnish

SAUCE: Place the ingredients in a blender and puree until smooth, about 1 minute. Set aside.

BURRITOS: Preheat the oven to 350 degrees. Lay a tortilla on your working surface. Spoon about ¼ cup black beans across the center of the tortilla, followed by a tablespoon each of onion, rice, and cheese. Roll up and place the burrito seam side down in a 9-by-13-inch lightly oiled baking dish. Repeat with the remaining tortillas, onion, rice, and cheese.

Spoon the sauce over the burritos and bake for 12 minutes. Serve the burritos topped with the sour cream, avocado if using, and cilantro.

PER SERVING: 357 calories; 18g protein; 56g carbohydrates; 8g fat (21 percent calories from fat); 6g fiber; 17mg cholesterol; 418mg sodium.

Mushroom-Onion-Tomato Pizza

This pizza is simple to prepare, thanks to the bread dough crust. You can find bread dough in supermarket freezers.

1 pound frozen bread dough, thawed
Cornmeal for dusting
½ tablespoon virgin olive oil
1 onion, chopped
1½ cups sliced crimini mushrooms
2 to 4 tablespoons sun-dried tomatoes packed in oil, drained and blotted dry

⅓ to ½ cup Quick Marinara Sauce (page 255) or your favorite pasta sauce
1 cup shredded part-skim mozzarella cheese

MAKES 8; SERVES 4

Shape the dough into a ball and roll out on your work surface into a 12- to 14-inch circle. Sprinkle a light dusting of cornmeal onto a pizza pan or a baking sheet. Place the dough circle on top. Set aside.

Heat the oil in a skillet over medium heat and sauté the onion, mushrooms, and tomatoes until the onion is limp, about 10 minutes.

Preheat the oven to 400 degrees. Spread the sauce on the dough circle. Arrange the mushroom mixture on top. Sprinkle with the cheese. Bake until the cheese is melted and the crust is lightly browned, about 15 minutes. Cut into eight pieces and serve.

PER SERVING: 398 calories; 17g protein; 61g carbohydrates; 10g fat (23 percent calories from fat); 4g fiber; 16mg cholesterol; 768mg sodium.

The Best Macaroni-and-Cheese Casserole

This slimmed-down comfort food delivers B vitamins, calcium, selenium, and, of course, a walk down memory lane.

2 cups uncooked macaroni
3 tablespoons reduced-fat
   margarine or butter
¼ cup onion, diced
½ teaspoon salt
¼ white pepper
½ to 1 teaspoon ground mustard
1¼ cups reduced-fat soymilk or
   skim milk, warmed

½ cup low-fat small-curd cottage
   cheese
¾ to 1 cup reduced-fat sharp
   cheddar cheese
¼ cup dry bread crumbs,
   preferably whole wheat
2 tablespoons freshly grated
   Parmesan cheese

SERVES 4

Prepare the macaroni according to the package directions; drain. Meanwhile, in a large saucepan, melt 2 tablespoons of the margarine or butter over medium heat. Sauté the onion until transparent, about 7 minutes. Stir in the salt, pepper, and mustard. Remove from the heat. Add the macaroni to the saucepan along with the milk.

Preheat the oven to 350 degrees. Lightly oil a 2-quart casserole dish and spoon in the macaroni mixture. In a medium bowl, mix together the cheeses until smooth. Add to the casserole and toss.

In a small bowl, mix together the bread crumbs, Parmesan, and the remaining 1 tablespoon margarine or butter with your fingers. Sprinkle on top of the casserole. Bake until bubbly and lightly browned, about 30 minutes. Let stand 10 minutes before serving.

> PER SERVING: 349 calories; 19g protein; 44g carbohydrates; 13g fat (33 percent calories from fat); 2g fiber; 24mg cholesterol; 786mg sodium.

■ STRESS BUSTERS ■

Tense, uptight, or jittery? These carbo-packed, low-protein stress busters help get the amino acid tryptophan to your brain to make the "comforting" neurotransmitter serotonin. They're easy on fat and rich in a slew of vitamins (the

HIGH–VITAMIN B_{12} FOODS

Fortified cereal
Low-fat cottage cheese
Yogurt
Whole or skim milk
Whole egg
Ricotta cheese
Cheese

B's, especially thiamine, riboflavin, B_6, pantothenic acid, and folic acid; and C) and minerals (potassium, magnesium, iron, and selenium). Sugar is okay in moderation if eaten with complex carbos. So is chocolate.

Buttermilk Pancakes with Fruit Toppings

These pancakes are the best I've ever eaten. I often make them for dinner, for my mornings are already busy getting the kids off to school.

PANCAKES:

½ cup rolled oats
1½ cups unbleached white flour
½ cup whole-wheat flour
3 tablespoons granulated sugar
1 tablespoon baking powder
2 teaspoons baking soda

¾ teaspoon salt
2 eggs, separated (or 2 egg whites)
1 tablespoon canola or safflower oil
2 cups buttermilk

TOPPING 1:

1 cup fresh or frozen blueberries
¼ cup apple juice

1 tablespoon arrowroot dissolved in 2 tablespoons apple juice

TOPPING 2:

1 cup fresh or frozen sliced strawberries
¼ cup orange juice

1 tablespoon arrowroot dissolved in 2 tablespoons orange juice

TOPPING 3:

1 cup fresh or frozen peaches
¼ cup pear or apple juice

1 tablespoon arrowroot dissolved in 2 tablespoons pear or apple juice

SERVES 4

PANCAKES: In a blender, pulverize the rolled oats into a flour. Combine this oat flour with the other flours, sugar, baking powder, baking soda, and salt. In another bowl, blend the yolks if using, oil, and buttermilk. In a small bowl, beat the egg whites with an electric mixer until they make stiff peaks. (You may skip this step, but your pancakes will be fluffier if you take the few extra minutes to beat the whites.) Add the butter-milk mixture to the dry ingredients, blending until just moistened. Fold in the egg whites.

Heat a nonstick griddle on medium-high until a little water dropped on the surface dances. Reduce the heat to medium. For each pancake, ladle about ¼ cup of the batter onto the griddle. Cook until the underside browns nicely, about 3 or 4 minutes. Flip with a spatula and cook the other side about 2 minutes more. Place the pancakes on a plate in a 200-degree oven to keep them warm as you cook the remaining pancakes and make the toppings.

HIGH–PANTOTHENIC ACID FOODS
Whole egg
Broccoli
Whole or skim milk
Sweet potato
Molasses
Corn
Lentils
Peanuts
Peas
Soybeans
Sunflower seeds
Wheat germ
Whole-grain flour
Blue cheese

TOPPINGS: To make any of the toppings, chop the fruit (except blueberries) and place in a small saucepan with the fruit juice over medium-low heat, stirring frequently, until warmed, about 10 minutes. Increase the heat to medium-high, and gradually pour in the arrowroot-juice mixture. Stir frequently. Once the topping reaches desired thickness, remove from the heat. Serve warm with the pancakes.

PER SERVING: 435 calories; 16g protein; 73g carbohydrates; 8g fat (17 percent calories from fat); 5g fiber; 110mg cholesterol; 585 mg sodium.

Spinach Dip with Roasted Red Pepper in a Round Loaf

This dip mimics a perennial party favorite but is far lower in fat. If you're crunched for time, use a package of ranch-style dressing in place of the garlic, herbs, and spices, and opt for jarred roasted red peppers.

One 10-ounce package frozen chopped spinach, thawed
One 8-ounce can water chestnuts, drained and chopped
2 to 4 tablespoons diced red onion
⅔ cup nonfat sour cream
2 to 4 tablespoons nonfat or reduced-fat mayonnaise

1 tablespoon minced fresh garlic
2 teaspoons dried dill weed
½ teaspoon coriander powder
Dash cayenne pepper
Salt to taste
Up to 2 tablespoons buttermilk
One 1-pound round bread loaf
1 roasted red bell pepper, cored and chopped (see tip, below)

MAKES 1¾ CUPS OF DIP; SERVES 8

In a medium bowl, mix together the spinach, water chestnuts, and onion. In another bowl, combine the sour cream and mayonnaise. Stir the garlic, dill weed, coriander, cayenne, and salt into the sour cream mixture. Then add the spinach mixture and combine thoroughly. Add the buttermilk as needed to reach desired consistency. Chill at least 1 hour.

To prepare the bread loaf, cut a circle in its top about two inches smaller than the perimeter of the loaf using a serrated knife. Cut toward the bottom of the loaf, leaving about a 2-inch thickness. Remove chunks of bread. Cut the chunks into large, bite-size pieces. Place the hollowed-out loaf on a platter. Surround it with the bread pieces.

Just before serving, gently stir the red pepper into the spinach dip and spoon into the hollow of the loaf.

A Tip: To roast a bell pepper, hold it with tongs over a flame, such as a burner on a gas oven, until blackened all over. Place in a paper bag and let steam for 10 minutes. Remove from the bag and wipe off the charred skin with a paper towel.

PER SERVING: 175 calories; 8g protein; 33g carbohydrates; 2g fat (10 percent calories from fat); 6g fiber; 1mg cholesterol; 326mg sodium.

Salsa Fresca with Baked Tortilla Chips

This next-to-no-fat snack is not *muy caliente.* In other words, it won't burn your mouth. It's got beta-carotene, vitamin C, fiber, and phytochemicals.

6 to 8 fresh plum tomatoes, chopped and placed in a colander to drain

4 scallions (white and green parts), sliced

2 to 4 tablespoons chopped green bell pepper

2 teaspoons minced fresh garlic

2 tablespoons chopped fresh cilantro leaves or fresh parsley leaves

2 tablespoons minced green chilies, canned or fresh, seeded

6 corn tortillas, cut or torn into triangles and baked at 325 degrees on baking sheets until crisp, about 30 minutes (or use 6 cups store-bought baked, not fried, tortilla chips)

Serves 6

In a bowl, combine all of the ingredients except the tortilla chips. Let chill for at least 1 hour. To serve, transfer the salsa to a serving dish and place the tortilla chips on a platter.

PER SERVING: 95 calories; 3g protein; 21g carbohydrates; 1g fat (10 percent calories from fat); 4g fiber; 0mg cholesterol; 146mg sodium.

Vegetable Paella

In Spain this dish piles on short-grain paella rice, but Italian Arborio works well too. It marries with the artichokes, fennel, peas, and other vegetables for a feast for the eyes and the appetite.

1 tablespoon virgin olive oil
1 onion, chopped
1 tablespoon minced fresh garlic
1 cup chopped fennel bulb (see tips, below)
1 cup uncooked Arborio rice
One 14½-ounce can stewed tomatoes with liquid
2 cups Basic Vegetable Stock (page 247)
¼ cup dry white wine
½ to 1 teaspoon saffron threads (see tips, below)

One 14-ounce can quartered artichoke hearts, drained
1 red bell pepper, cored and chopped
1 cup frozen green peas, thawed
One 15-ounce can chickpeas, rinsed and drained (optional)
Salt to taste
Generous splash of cayenne pepper sauce, or to taste
Chopped fresh cilantro for garnish

SERVES 6

In a large saucepan, heat the oil over medium-high heat. Sauté the onion and garlic until the onion is softened, about 5 minutes. Reduce the heat to medium, add the fennel, and cook 5 minutes more. Stir in the rice, stewed tomatoes with liquid, vegetable stock, wine, and saffron. Bring to a boil, stirring occasionally, over medium-high heat.

Meanwhile, measure out 1 cup artichoke hearts and chop them coarsely. Add to the saucepan with the red bell pepper, cover, and simmer over medium-low heat until most of the liquid is absorbed, about 15 minutes. Stir in the peas, chickpeas if using, and salt. Cover, remove from the heat, and let stand until the liquid is absorbed, about 5 to 10 minutes more. Season with the cayenne pepper sauce. Transfer the paella to a platter and garnish with the cilantro. Serve warm.

A Few Tips: Fennel is a deliciously mild root vegetable that often shows up in soup. Its fronds have a strong licorice taste. If you're a licorice aficionado, then garnish this dish with the fronds too.

Saffron is an expensive yet absolutely essential spice for paella. The threads are the least expensive form. Look for them in well-stocked supermarkets or ethnic groceries.

> PER SERVING: 181 calories; 5g protein; 34g carbohydrates; 3g fat (15 percent calories from fat); 5g fiber; 0mg cholesterol; 318mg sodium.

Spicy Sesame Noodles

I could eat pasta every day—especially udon and soba noodles. This haute Asian fusion dish uses soba. You can find soba noodles at large supermarkets, natural food stores, or Asian markets.

1 pound whole-wheat soba noodles or regular linguine
1 tablespoon sesame oil (see tip, on page 278)
6 scallions (green parts only), sliced
1 red bell pepper, sliced
1 teaspoon peeled and minced gingerroot

½ cup fresh cilantro leaves
½ teaspoon cayenne pepper, or to taste
2 teaspoons low-sodium soy sauce or shoyu, or to taste
¼ cup toasted sesame seeds

SERVES 6

Prepare the noodles according to the package directions. Drain. Transfer to a serving dish. Cover.

In a medium skillet, heat the oil over medium-high heat and sauté the scallions, red bell pepper, and gingerroot for 2 minutes. Add the cilantro, cayenne, and soy sauce or shoyu, and sauté a minute more. Toss with the noodles. Sprinkle the sesame seeds on top. Serve warm or cold.

A Tip: Sesame oil has a distinctive, appealing flavor. Toasted sesame oil has a stronger, earthier flavor. If it's your favorite, by all means use it.

PER SERVING: 331 calories; 14g protein; 57g carbohydrates; 7g fat (18 percent calories from fat); 4g fiber; 0mg cholesterol; 69mg sodium.

Capellini Pomodoro

This wonderful dish that I like to serve to company has an earthy yet light flavor. A good stock is essential.

1 tablespoon virgin olive oil
1 Vidalia or other sweet onion, chopped
8 white button mushrooms, chopped
8 plum tomatoes, seeded and chopped
¼ cup chopped Kalamata olives

½ cup Basic Vegetable Stock (page 247)
2 or 3 drops cayenne pepper sauce (or ¼ teaspoon cayenne pepper), or to taste
1 pound uncooked angel hair pasta
¼ cup chopped fresh oregano

SERVES 4

In a small saucepan, heat the olive oil over medium-high, swirling the pan to coat the bottom. Lower the heat to medium. Add the onion and mushrooms and sauté until barely limp, about 6 minutes. Stir in the tomatoes and olives and cook 3 minutes more. Add the remaining ingredients except the pasta and oregano and cook for 5 minutes.

Meanwhile, cook the pasta according to the package directions; drain. Transfer the pasta to a serving dish. Pour the sauce on top and toss to coat. Garnish with the oregano. Serve at once.

> PER SERVING: 359 calories; 14g protein; 63g carbohydrates; 7g fat (18 percent calories from fat); 5g fiber; 0mg cholesterol; 368mg sodium.

Mediterranean Pasta

Gemelli is a type of corkscrew pasta. If you don't have it on hand, use another favorite. The trio of greens, feta, and sun-dried tomatoes is common to the cuisine of Crete.

½ pound uncooked gemelli
1 recipe Greens Sauté with
    Fennel (page 340), warmed
½ cup crumbled feta cheese

2 tablespoons chopped sun-dried
    tomatoes packed in oil,
    drained, for garnish

SERVES 6

Prepare the pasta according to package directions; drain. Transfer to a serving dish. Toss with the sauté, top with the feta, and garnish with the tomatoes.

> PER SERVING: 278 calories; 11g protein; 43g carbohydrates; 7g fat (23 percent calories from fat); 3g fiber; 17mg cholesterol; 580mg sodium.

Potato Pierogi and Vegetable Sauté

Pierogi is a traditional Polish dish served with enough butter to cause cardiac arrest. This update goes very easy on the fat and heavy on vitamin-packed additions.

One 16- to 20-ounce package
    frozen potato-filled pierogies
2 teaspoons canola or safflower
    oil
½ onion, thinly sliced
¾ cup Basic Vegetable Stock
    (page 247)

One 1-pound package vegetable
    stir-fry blend of choice (see
    tip, below)
2 tablespoons chopped fresh
    parsley
Freshly ground black pepper to
    taste

SERVES 4

Cook the pierogies according to package directions; rinse, drain, and transfer to a serving platter.

In a large saucepan, heat the oil over medium-high heat, swirling the pan to coat. Sauté the onion, stirring frequently, for 3 or 4 minutes. Reduce the heat to medium. Pour in the stock and add the stir-fry; cover. Let simmer until the vegetables are warmed through, about 8 minutes. Uncover and simmer another 1 or 2 minutes. Spoon the vegetables on top of the pierogies. Sprinkle the parsley and black pepper on top. Serve warm.

A Tip: Many varieties of stir-fry blends fill the supermarkets' freezers. Choose the one that strikes your fancy.

PER SERVING: 196 calories; 7g protein; 35g carbohydrates; 4g fat (18 percent calories from fat); 6g fiber; 3mg cholesterol; 429mg sodium.

Crimini-and-Apricot-Stuffed Crepes with Rich Gravy

Don't let the word *crepe* unnerve you. This easy-to-prepare, sweet-savory dish is loaded with calming carbos and vitamins.

CREPES:

1 egg
⅔ cup reduced-fat soymilk or skim milk

½ cup unbleached white flour
Dash salt

STUFFING:

2 teaspoons butter (or canola or safflower oil)
1 onion, chopped
⅔ cup chopped crimini mushrooms or white button mushrooms
⅔ cup uncooked bulgur (see tip, below)

1 cup Basic Vegetable Stock (page 247)
⅓ cup chopped dried apricots
2 tablespoons chopped, toasted pecans
Salt and freshly ground black pepper to taste

GRAVY:

2 teaspoons canola or safflower oil
½ onion, diced
½ teaspoon minced fresh garlic
½ cup whole-wheat flour
2 cups Basic Vegetable Stock (page 247)

2 to 4 tablespoons low-sodium soy sauce or tamari
Freshly ground black pepper to taste

MAKES 8; SERVES 4

CREPES: Combine the crepe ingredients in a blender or food processor and whirl until smooth. Transfer to a bowl. Let stand 30 minutes.

STUFFING: In a large saucepan, heat the butter or oil over medium heat. Sauté the onion and mushrooms until the onion is transparent, about 10 minutes. Add the bulgur and vegetable stock and bring to a boil over medium-high heat. Cover, reduce heat to medium-low, and simmer 20 to 30 minutes. Stir in the apricots, pecans, salt, and pepper. Remove from the heat.

GRAVY: In a medium saucepan, heat the oil over medium-high heat. (Do this while the stuffing mixture is simmering.) Sauté the onion and garlic until the onion is transparent, about 5 minutes. Gradually blend in the flour and cook until lightly toasted, about 2 minutes. Slowly add the vegetable stock, stirring constantly. Add the soy sauce or tamari and pepper and cook, stirring frequently, until thickened, about 5 minutes. Transfer to a serving bowl.

To make and assemble the crepes, lightly oil an 8-inch nonstick skillet. Heat over medium heat. Pour 2 or 3 tablespoons of the batter into the center of the skillet, tilting it gently so the batter spreads to the edges. Cook 30 to 40 seconds. Loosen an edge of the crepe with a spatula and flip over. Cook 15 seconds more. Slide the crepe onto a sheet of waxed paper. Repeat this procedure until all of the batter is used up, stacking the crepes between sheets of waxed paper.

Place a crepe on a plate and spread about 3 tablespoons of the stuffing over half of the crepe and fold the crepe over. Transfer to a serving dish. Repeat with the remaining crepes and stuffing.

Pass the gravy for diners to spoon over their crepes.

A Tip: Bulgur is a nutty-flavored, quick-cooking grain sold in natural food stores and most supermarkets.

PER SERVING: 312 calories; 11g protein; 50g carbohydrates; 9g fat (25 percent calories from fat); 9g fiber; 59mg cholesterol; 467mg sodium.

Sweet Peppers Stuffed with Seasoned Bulgur

Bulgur combines with onions and herbs to fill lovely-colored peppers. This dish is high in beta-carotene, vitamin C, and fiber.

3 bell peppers (1 each of red, yellow, and green), halved and seeded
2 teaspoons butter or reduced-fat margarine
1 cup chopped Spanish onion
½ cup chopped celery
1 teaspoon dried marjoram
½ teaspoon poultry seasoning or sage

1½ cups uncooked bulgur
2½ cups Basic Vegetable Stock (page 247)
3 tablespoons grated fresh Parmesan cheese
6 tablespoons dry bread crumbs, preferably whole wheat
Salt and freshly ground black pepper to taste

SERVES 3

Bring a large pot of water to boil. Gently drop in the pepper halves and cook until barely tender, about 5 minutes. Remove and invert on paper towels to cool.

In a large saucepan, melt the butter or margarine over medium heat and sauté the onion until transparent, about 10 minutes. Add the celery and seasonings and cook 5 minutes more. Stir in the bulgur and vegetable stock. Increase the heat to medium-high, bring to a boil, cover, and reduce the heat to medium-low. Simmer until the liquid is absorbed, about 20 minutes. Remove from the heat.

Preheat the oven to 350 degrees. Snuggle the pepper halves, cut sides up, in a lightly oiled baking pan, so they don't tip. Fill each with the bulgur mixture. Sprinkle ½ tablespoon cheese and 1 tablespoon bread crumbs on each stuffed pepper. Season with the salt and black pepper. Bake until warmed through, about 25 minutes. Serve hot.

PER SERVING: 370 calories; 14g protein; 71g carbohydrates; 6g fat (14 percent calories from fat); 16g fiber; 11mg cholesterol; 271mg sodium.

Strawberry Muffins

These almost fat-free muffins are just sweet enough and have pretty peaks.

¾ cup finely chopped
   strawberries
2 teaspoons honey
2 cups unbleached white flour
1 cup whole-wheat flour
½ cup granulated sugar

1½ teaspoons baking powder
¾ teaspoon baking soda
1½ cups buttermilk
4 egg whites or 2 eggs, lightly
   beaten

Makes 12

Preheat the oven to 500 degrees. Place the strawberries in a bowl and toss with the honey. Set aside.

In a large bowl, combine the flours, sugar, baking powder, and baking soda. In a large measuring cup or a medium bowl, mix together the buttermilk and egg whites or eggs. Stir in the strawberries. Pour into the dry ingredients and gently stir until just moistened.

Fill the cups of a lightly oiled, nonstick 12-cup muffin tin. Place in the oven and reduce temperature to 400 degrees. Bake until a toothpick inserted in the middle of a muffin comes out clean, about 20 to 25 minutes.

Smart Note: Don't use paper liners with fat-free muffins; they'll stick. For a taste change, replace the strawberries with another fresh fruit. Peaches, apricots, and, of course, blueberries work wonderfully.

PER SERVING: 162 calories; 6g protein; 33g carbohydrates; 1g fat (6 percent calories from fat); 2g fiber; 1mg cholesterol; 190mg sodium.

Nutty Apricot Muffins

Another delicious snack for calming down. Try one an hour before bedtime to help you sleep easy.

2 cups unbleached white flour
1 cup whole-wheat flour
⅔ cup granulated sugar
1½ teaspoons baking powder
¾ teaspoon baking soda
½ cup finely chopped dried
   apricots

⅓ cup finely chopped pecans,
   Brazil nuts, or toasted
   almonds
1¾ cups buttermilk
2 eggs or 4 eggs white lightly
   beaten

MAKES 12

Preheat the oven to 500 degrees. In a large bowl, combine the flours, sugar, baking powder, and baking soda. Stir in the apricots and nuts. In a large measuring cup or a medium bowl, mix together the buttermilk and egg whites or eggs. Pour into the dry ingredients and gently stir until just moistened.

Fill the cups of a lightly oiled, nonstick 12-cup muffin tin. Place in oven and reduce temperature to 400 degrees. Bake until a toothpick inserted in the middle of a muffin comes out clean, about 20 to 25 minutes.

Smart Note: Change the flavor by varying the nuts and dried fruit. Try pecans with dried cranberries, toasted almonds with dried cherries, or walnuts with chopped raisins.

PER SERVING: 204 calories; 6g protein; 37g carbohydrates; 4g fat (18 percent calories from fat); 2g fiber; 37mg cholesterol; 188mg sodium.

Apple Cinnamon Bread

This treat, like other grain-based dishes, boasts B vitamins, which help make the "comforting" neurotransmitter serotonin.

2 cups unbleached white flour
1 cup whole-wheat flour
⅔ cup granulated sugar
1 teaspoon ground cinnamon
1½ teaspoons baking powder

¾ teaspoon baking soda
1¾ cups buttermilk
2 eggs, lightly beaten
⅔ cup finely diced apple
Confectioners' sugar (optional)

SERVES 16

Preheat the oven to 400 degrees. In a large bowl, combine the flours, sugar, cinnamon, baking powder, and baking soda. In a large measuring cup or a medium bowl, mix together the buttermilk, eggs, and apple. Pour into the dry ingredients and gently stir until just moistened.

Pour the batter into a lightly oiled, nonstick 8-inch-square baking pan.

> **HIGH–FOLIC ACID FOODS**
>
> Barley
> Legumes
> Endive
> Fruits
> Green leafy vegetables
> Brown rice
> Soybeans
> Sprouts
> Wheat germ

Bake until a toothpick inserted in the middle comes out clean, about 20 minutes. Let cool. Sprinkle with Confectioners' sugar if using.

PER SERVING: 134 calories; 4g protein; 26g carbohydrates; 1g fat (8 percent calories from fat); 1g fiber; 28mg cholesterol; 141mg sodium.

Strawberry Orange Ice

This refreshing meal-ender or snack is a pretty, deep pink, and it's flavorful and vitamin-rich.

1 cup calcium-fortified orange
    juice
2 cups strawberries, fresh or
    frozen, pureed

1 tablespoon fresh lemon juice
¼ cup granulated sugar
Orange slices for garnish

SERVES 4

In a large bowl, combine all the ingredients except for the orange slices. Pour into a shallow, nonmetallic pan and freeze, stirring occasionally, until almost frozen, about 3 or so hours. (Freezing time depends on the shallowness of the container and the temperature of the freezer.) Spoon into four dessert dishes, garnish with the orange slices, and serve at once.

PER SERVING: 104 calories; 0g protein; 26g carbohydrates; 0g fat (0 percent calories from fat); 2g fiber; 0mg cholesterol; 8mg sodium.

Gingery Lemon Ice

Just sweet enough, this summer favorite delivers vitamins along with flavor. Be sure to use fresh lemon juice; the bottled stuff can't do this dish justice.

½ cup granulated sugar
½ cup water
1 to 2 tablespoons peeled and
    chopped gingerroot

1 cup fresh lemon juice
Lemon slices for garnish

SERVES 4

In a medium saucepan over medium-low heat, simmer the sugar and water, stirring occasionally until the sugar is dissolved, about 10 minutes. Remove from the heat. Stir in the gingerroot and let stand, covered, for 20 minutes. Add the lemon juice.

Pour into a shallow, nonmetallic pan and freeze, stirring occasionally, until frozen, about 3 or so hours. Divide among four dessert dishes. Garnish with the lemon slices. Serve at once.

PER SERVING: 108 calories; 0g protein; 29g carbohydrates; 0g fat (0 percent calories from fat); 0g fiber; 0mg cholesterol; 1mg sodium.

▪ MOOD ENHANCERS ▪

A mood boost is as simple as a carbo-loaded pie or pilaf or pretzel. Eating carbos helps speed the amino acid tryptophan to the brain, where it can manufacture the neurotransmitter serotonin. Steer clear of heavy protein and fat, which interfere with serotonin production. Mood enhancers also are rich in the B vitamins, especially thiamine, riboflavin, B, pantothenic acid, and folic acid, and the mineral selenium. Sugar and chocolate are perfectly acceptable in moderation.

HIGH–VITAMIN C FOODS

Papaya
Guava
Strawberries
Kiwifruit
Cantaloupe
Broccoli
Brussels sprouts
Grapefruit
Potato
Pineapple
Cabbage
Tomato
Blueberries

Not Quite Champagne

This drink tastes light and festive—and amazingly like the real thing. It's a favorite among my cooking classes, so I make extra.

Two 2-liter bottles plain seltzer
Four 6-ounce cans frozen white
    grape juice, thawed

¼ cup cranberry juice or
    grenadine

SERVES 16

In a pitcher, very gently stir together all the ingredients. Serve at once in champagne glasses or keep chilled and very well covered until serving time.

> PER SERVING: 78 calories; 1g protein; 19g carbohydrates; 0g fat (0 percent calories from fat); 0g fiber; 0mg cholesterol; 4mg sodium.

Banana Walnut Muffins

Halve your muffin, spoon on all-fruit spread, and enjoy.

1 cup whole-wheat flour
1½ cups unbleached white
    flour
¾ cup granulated sugar
1½ teaspoons baking powder
1 teaspoon baking soda
¾ teaspoon salt
2 tablespoons reduced-fat
    margarine

2 tablespoons unsweetened
    applesauce
1 cup mashed banana (see tips,
    below)
⅔ cup buttermilk, sour milk (see
    tips, below), or reduced-fat
    soymilk
2 eggs or ½ cup egg substitute
1 teaspoon vanilla extract

MAKES 12

Preheat the oven to 350 degrees. Lightly oil a 12-muffin tin. In a large mixing bowl, combine the flours, sugar, baking powder, baking soda, and salt. Add the margarine, applesauce, and banana, and mix with an electric beater on low speed until combined.

Add the remaining ingredients. Beat on high speed, scraping the sides of the bowl occasionally, for 2 minutes. Spoon into the muffin tins. Bake until lightly browned, about 15 minutes.

A Few Tips: A mess-free method of mashing bananas is to place them in a ziplock plastic baggie, close tightly, and mash, using your fingers.

To make sour milk, pour 2 tablespoons of white distilled vinegar into a measuring cup and add milk to measure ⅔ cup.

PER SERVING: 184 calories; 5g protein; 36g carbohydrates; 3g fat (15 percent calories from fat); 2g fiber; 36mg cholesterol; 356mg sodium.

Carrot Bran Muffins

These treats make a great breakfast or anytime snack.

1 cup crushed bran flakes cereal
1 cup unbleached white flour
½ cup whole-wheat flour
¼ cup packed brown sugar
2 teaspoons baking powder
½ teaspoon baking soda
1 teaspoon ground cinnamon
¼ teaspoon ground nutmeg

1¼ cups reduced-fat soymilk or
skim milk
1 egg, beaten
3 tablespoons canola or safflower
oil
1½ cups grated carrots
1½ cup crushed pineapple, well-
drained

MAKES 18

Preheat the oven to 400 degrees. Lightly oil 18 nonstick muffin cups. In a large bowl, combine the dry ingredients. Make a well in the center. Pour in the soymilk or skim milk, egg, and oil. Blend until just combined. Gently stir in the carrots and pineapple. Bake for 45 minutes.

> PER SERVING: 99 calories; 3g protein; 17g carbohydrates; 3g fat (26 percent calories from fat); 2g fiber; 12mg cholesterol; 141mg sodium.

Blueberry Sour Cream Scones

Scones are sweet biscuits, pure and simple. They are traditionally made with cream, butter, and eggs. This version relies on oats for a subtle buttery flavor, nonfat sour cream for moistness, and blueberry preserves for sweetness.

1 cup rolled oats
1 cup unbleached white flour
4 teaspoons baking power
½ teaspoon baking soda
½ teaspoon salt

¼ teaspoon ground nutmeg
¾ cup nonfat sour cream
⅓ cup egg substitute or 1 egg
½ cup blueberry preserves

MAKES 12

Preheat the oven to 400 degrees. Lightly oil a baking sheet. In a blender, pulverize the oats to make a flour. Combine the flours, baking powder, baking soda, salt, and nutmeg. In another bowl, beat together the sour cream and egg substitute or egg. Make a well in the center of the dry ingredients, and add the sour cream mixture, mixing with swift strokes, until just blended.

HIGH–VITAMIN E FOODS
Almonds
Corn oil
Cottonseed oil
Filberts
Peanut oil
Safflower oil
Sunflower oil
Sunflower seeds
Walnuts
Wheat germ
Whole-grain flour

Drop by rounded quarter-cup measures onto the prepared

baking sheet. Gently poke the centers. Dollop 2 teaspoons preserves into the indentation on each scone. Bake about 12 to 15
minutes. Serve warm.

Variation: Feel free to substitute your favorite preserves for the
blueberry. Good bets are apricot, strawberry, and raspberry.

> PER SERVING: 107 calories; 3g protein; 22g carbohydrates; 1g fat (8
> percent calories from fat); 1g fiber; 1mg cholesterol; 324mg sodium.

Fruity Couscous Salad

This quick-cooking Moroccan grain has a mild nutty flavor that
suits dried fruits and aromatic spices.

1½ cups Basic Vegetable Stock
  (page 247) or water
1 cup uncooked couscous,
  preferably whole-wheat
3 tablespoons calcium-fortified
  orange juice
1 tablespoon virgin olive oil
1 tablespoon chopped fresh
  cilantro (optional)
½ teaspoon ground cinnamon
Dash salt

½ cup dried sweetened
  cranberries
½ cup golden raisins
2 scallions (green and white
  parts), diced
2 celery stalks, minced
Lettuce
3 tablespoons chopped pecans or
  other nut, for garnish

Serves 4

In a small pot over medium-high heat, bring the vegetable stock
or water to a boil. Stir in the couscous, remove from heat, and
cover with a tight-fitting lid. Let stand 5 minutes.

Combine the juice, olive oil, cilantro if using, cinnamon, and
salt. Transfer the couscous to a serving bowl, and pour the juice-
oil mixture on top. Toss with a fork. Add the cranberries, raisins,
scallions, and celery, and toss again. Let cool.

Line four plates with lettuce. Mound the couscous salad on top. Garnish with the nuts.

PER SERVING: 308 calories; 7g protein; 55g carbohydrates; 7g fat (21 percent calories from fat); 5g fiber; 0mg cholesterol; 146mg sodium.

Crostini with Tomatoes, Kalamata Olives, and Basil

Crostini are bite-sized Italian toasts adorned simply with olive oil and herbs or dressed up, as they are here. Traditionally, chopped liver tops crostini.

1 small loaf baguette-style bread
½ cup nonfat or part-skim
    ricotta cheese
3 plum tomatoes, seeded, diced,
    and set over a colander to
    drain
¼ cup Kalamata olives, minced

2 tablespoons diced onion
⅓ cup chopped fresh basil leaves
1 tablespoon balsamic vinegar
1 teaspoon minced fresh garlic
Salt and freshly ground black
    pepper to taste

MAKES 24; SERVES 6

Preheat the oven to 350 degrees. Slice the bread into twenty-four one-quarter-inch slices. Flatten the slices with a rolling pin. Cut out circles or other shape with a cookie cutter. Place the bread in a single layer on a baking sheet and toast in oven for just a couple of minutes. Set aside.

In a blender, process the remaining ingredients until very well combined, about 10 seconds. Spread on the toasts. Serve.

PER SERVING: 226 calories; 11g protein; 39g carbohydrates; 2g fat (8 percent calories from fat); 2g fiber; 1mg cholesterol; 562mg sodium.

Cucumber Party Sandwiches

My sister-in-law, Mary, perfected this buffet favorite with a few fat-free switcheroos. Serve it as a snack, with fruit for a light lunch, or as great party food.

One 8-ounce container nonfat cream cheese
1 small package of Italian dressing mix
1 tablespoon nonfat mayonnaise or plain yogurt

1 loaf cocktail rye bread
2 cucumbers, peeled and sliced thinly
2 tablespoons fresh dill (or 2 teaspoons dried)

SERVES 8

In a bowl, combine the cream cheese, Italian dressing mix, and mayonnaise or yogurt until well blended. Spread over the bread and top with cucumber slices. Sprinkle with the dill.

PER SERVING: 175 calories; 9g protein; 34g carbohydrates; 0g fat (0 percent calories from fat); 4g fiber; 1mg cholesterol; 468mg sodium.

Garden Vegetable Wrap

Wraps are popular because they're easy to tote, hold, and eat, and are stuffed with an amazing number of fillings. This one goes for a vitamin crunch.

Four 8-inch flour tortillas, preferably whole wheat
4 slices reduced-fat Swiss cheese (optional)
4 leaves romaine lettuce
1 cup grated carrot
1 cup grated zucchini
4 scallions, slivered lengthwise
½ avocado, peeled, pitted, and sliced
1 cup adzuki bean sprouts or other favorite sprouts

2 tablespoons sunflower seeds
2 tablespoons raisins
2 tablespoons chopped fresh tarragon leaves
2 tablespoons rice vinegar mixed with 1 tablespoon Dijon-style mustard
Salt and freshly ground black pepper to taste
Cayenne pepper to taste

SERVES 4

Line each tortilla with a slice of cheese if using and a lettuce leaf. Divide the carrot, zucchini, scallions, and avocado among the tortillas. Top with the sprouts, seeds, raisins, and tarragon. Dribble the vinegar-mustard mixture over the tortillas and season with the salt, black pepper, and cayenne pepper.

Roll up each tortilla tightly, tucking in the sides as you roll. Cut in half. Serve at once or wrap in plastic wrap.

PER SERVING: 153 calories; 6g protein; 32g carbohydrates; 4g fat (24 percent calories from fat); 5g fiber; 0mg cholesterol; 285mg sodium.

Portobello Mushroom Burgers

Unique to portobello is its meaty flavor and smell once cooked. You'd almost swear you had a porterhouse in your broiler if you didn't know otherwise.

6 portobello caps, trimmed and gently rinsed
½ cup balsamic vinegar
2 teaspoons vegetarian Worcestershire sauce
Virgin olive oil for brushing

6 whole-wheat burger buns
6 leaves romaine lettuce
Dijon-style mustard
Other burger trimmings of choice (optional)

SERVES 6

Preheat the broiler. In a shallow baking dish, marinate the portobello caps in the vinegar and Worcestershire sauce for 10 minutes. Place them on the broiler, lightly brush with the olive oil, and broil 5 minutes each side.

Meanwhile, line the burger buns with the lettuce. Spread with the mustard and add trimmings, if using. Place the burgers on top of the buns. Serve hot.

PER SERVING: 167 calories; 7g protein; 30g carbohydrates; 3g fat (16 percent calories from fat); 5g fiber; 0mg cholesterol; 302mg sodium.

Vegetable Knishes

My favorite natural food store is Whole Foods Market. Along with attractive and tasty organic produce, bulk grains, and packaged goods are its ready-for-the-eatin' food counters. I got the idea for this recipe from one of the delectables I sampled—they love to give out samples—and ordered.

One 1-pound loaf frozen bread
dough, thawed
¼ cup chopped, lightly steamed
broccoli
1 medium carrot, slivered and
lightly steamed
1 cup frozen green peas, thawed

2 cups well-seasoned mashed
potatoes
2 tablespoons fresh thyme (or 1
teaspoon dried)
Salt and freshly ground black
pepper to taste

MAKES 10; SERVES 5

Divide the bread dough into 10 equal parts. Roll each into a ball. On a floured bread board or other clean surface, roll out the balls into 6-inch circles with a rolling pin. Set aside.

Preheat the oven to 375 degrees. Combine the vegetables and thyme in a medium bowl. Season with the salt and pepper. Spoon a couple tablespoons of the mixture onto the middle of each dough circle.

To make a knish, fold up one side of a dough circle so it almost covers half of the vegetable mixture. Fold up the other sides in a similar fashion, pinching to seal. You should have a small peek-a-boo opening on top. Repeat with the remaining dough circles and filling.

Place them on a baking sheet, and bake until golden brown, about 20 minutes. Serve warm.

PER SERVING: 339 calories; 11g protein; 62g carbohydrates; 6g fat (17 percent calories from fat); 6g fiber; 2mg cholesterol; 744mg sodium.

Penne in Porcini and Red Wine Sauce

This sauce reminds me of bolognese, with beef as its main ingredient, for the porcini are earthy and meaty.

1 to 2 ounces dried porcini
  mushrooms, thoroughly rinsed
1 tablespoon virgin olive oil
1 small onion, minced
½ teaspoon minced fresh garlic
½ teaspoon fresh sage (or a
  pinch of dried)
1 teaspoon fresh lemon juice
½ pound white button
  mushrooms, sliced

⅓ cup dry red wine
Salt and freshly ground black
  pepper to taste
1 pound uncooked penne
4 scallions (green and white
  parts), sliced
1 medium tomato, seeded and
  diced

SERVES 6

Soak the porcini in hot water to cover until softened, about 20 minutes. Drain, reserving the soaking liquid, and chop the mushrooms. Set aside.

In a large saucepan, heat the olive oil over medium-high heat, swirling the pan to coat the bottom. Add the onion and garlic and sauté until the onion is nearly translucent, about 5 minutes. Stir in the sage, lemon juice, white button mushrooms, and porcini, and cook another 5 minutes, stirring frequently.

Add 1 cup porcini soaking liquid and simmer briskly over high heat until the liquid is reduced to a glaze. Stir in the wine and reduce again. Season with the salt and pepper.

Meanwhile, prepare the penne according to the package directions; drain. Transfer to a large pasta bowl or serving platter. Pour on the sauce and toss gently. Garnish with the scallions and tomato.

PER SERVING: 334 calories; 11g protein; 61g carbohydrates; 4g fat (10 percent calories from fat); 4g fiber; 0mg cholesterol; 352mg sodium.

Bulgur with Peas, Raisins, and Pine Nuts

Bulgur, also called cracked wheat, is nutty-flavored, chewy (as long as you don't overcook it), and nutritious. It pairs well with peas, fruit, and nuts—almost anything, really.

1½ cups Basic Vegetable Stock (page 247)
1 cup uncooked bulgur
One 10-ounce package frozen green peas
1 teaspoon virgin olive oil

½ cup diced onion
1 teaspoon minced fresh garlic
½ teaspoon dried dill weed
Salt to taste
⅓ cup raisins
¼ cup pine nuts, lightly toasted

SERVES 4

In a large saucepan, bring the stock to a boil over medium-high heat. Stir in the bulgur and peas, cover, reduce the heat to medium-low, and let simmer for 15 minutes. Remove from the heat.

Meanwhile, in a small skillet, heat the oil over medium-high heat, swirling the pan to coat the bottom. Sauté the onion and garlic until the onion is transparent, about 7 minutes. Very gently stir into the bulgur along with the dill weed, salt, and raisins. Transfer to a serving dish and sprinkle the pine nuts on top. Serve warm.

HIGH-IRON FOODS

Black beans
Lentils
Nori
Quinoa
Spinach
Kidney beans
Bran cereal
Dried figs
Pumpkin seeds
Sesame seeds
Swiss chard
Lima beans
Blackstrap molasses
Dried prunes
Raisins
Bulgur
Dried apricots
Whole-wheat bread

PER SERVING: 282 calories; 11g protein; 50g carbohydrates; 7g fat (22 percent calories from fat); 12g fiber; 0mg cholesterol; 81mg sodium.

Spicy Oatmeal Cookies

Tops in flavor and low in fat, these cookies contain my secret ingredient: apple butter. Contrary to its name, apple butter has no butter. Its fat content is zero.

¼ cup apple butter, preferably unsweetened
⅔ cup granulated sugar
1 egg
2 tablespoons safflower or canola oil
½ teaspoon vanilla extract
1 cup unbleached white flour

1 cup quick-cooking rolled oats
½ teaspoon baking soda
½ teaspoon salt
1 teaspoon ground cinnamon
½ teaspoon ground cloves
½ cup raisins
⅓ cup chopped walnuts

MAKES 36; SERVES 12

Preheat the oven to 375 degrees. In a medium bowl, thoroughly combine the apple butter, sugar, egg, oil, and vanilla. In another bowl, combine the flour, oats, baking soda, salt, and spices. Stir the dry ingredients into the wet ingredients. Add the raisins and walnuts, and stir until combined.

> HIGH-ZINC FOODS
>
> Bran (wheat and rice)
> Egg yolk
> Blackstrap molasses
> Soybeans
> Sunflower seeds
> Wheat germ
> Whole-grain flour

Drop the batter by spoonfuls onto baking sheets. Bake for 8 minutes. Let cool on paper towels. Store the cookies in an airtight container.

PER SERVING: 199 calories; 4g protein; 36g carbohydrates; 5g fat (23 percent calories from fat); 2g fiber; 18mg cholesterol; 153mg sodium.

The Miracle Chocolate Chip Cookie

This is my all-time favorite cookie: chewy, chocolate-y, just sweet enough, and—surprise—very low in fat. It has 1 gram of fiber per serving too. You can make it even lower in fat by using half the butter or omitting it altogether, with scrumptious results.

3 tablespoons apple butter, preferably unsweetened
⅔ cup granulated sugar
1 egg
Up to 2 tablespoons melted butter
½ teaspoon vanilla extract
1 cup unbleached white flour

¼ cup whole-wheat flour or unbleached white flour
½ teaspoon baking soda
½ teaspoon salt
¾ cup semisweet chocolate chips
¼ cup chopped pecans

MAKES 36; SERVES 12

Preheat the oven to 375 degrees. In a medium bowl, thoroughly combine the apple butter, sugar, egg, melted butter, and vanilla. In another bowl, combine the flours, baking soda, and salt. Stir the dry ingredients into the wet ingredients. Add the chocolate chips and pecans, and stir until combined.

Drop the batter by spoonfuls onto baking sheets. Bake for 8 minutes. Let cool on paper towels. Store the cookies in an airtight container.

Variation: For Chocolate Chip Oatmeal Cookies, replace ½ cup of the flour with quick-cooking rolled oats and proceed with the recipe as directed.

PER SERVING: 171 calories; 3g protein; 30g carbohydrates; 5g fat (26 percent calories from fat); 1g fiber; 18mg cholesterol; 154mg sodium.

Cranberry-Apple Crisp

This sweet-tart dessert is a serotonin-enhancing bonanza: It combines fruit, oats, spices, and just a smidgeon of fat.

⅔ cup dried sweetened
　cranberries
4 large Granny Smith apples,
　peeled and sliced thickly
¼ cup orange juice
¼ cup rolled oats
¼ cup unbleached white flour or
　whole-wheat flour

¼ cup firmly packed brown
　sugar
1 teaspoon ground cinnamon
½ teaspoon ground allspice
Dash ground nutmeg
1 tablespoon reduced-fat
　margarine or butter

SERVES 6

Preheat the oven to 375 degrees. In a medium bowl, combine the cranberries, apples, and juice. Transfer to a lightly oiled 8-inch square baking dish. In another bowl, stir together the oats, flour, sugar, and spices. Using your fingers, incorporate the butter or margarine until the mixture becomes crumbly. Sprinkle over the cranberry-apple mixture. Cover and bake 30 minutes, then uncover and bake 10 minutes more.

PER SERVING: 155 calories; 1g protein; 35g carbohydrates; 2g fat (12 percent calories from fat); 4g fiber; 0mg cholesterol; 26mg sodium.

Raspberry Cheese Crumb Cake

This dessert tastes far richer than its nutritional breakdown reveals.

TOPPING:

¾ cup rolled oats
¾ cup unbleached white or
   whole-wheat flour

½ cup packed brown sugar
Dash ground nutmeg
2 tablespoons butter

CAKE:

8 ounces fresh or frozen thawed
   raspberries
4 tablespoons frozen orange-juice
   concentrate, thawed
2 tablespoons cornstarch
A few tablespoons granulated
   sugar (optional)
½ cup farmer's cheese
½ cup nonfat sour cream

2 cups unbleached white flour
⅔ cup granulated sugar
1½ teaspoons baking powder
1 teaspoon baking soda
½ teaspoon salt
3 tablespoons butter, melted
½ cup egg substitute
2 teaspoons vanilla extract
1 cup buttermilk

Serves 16

TOPPING: In a medium bowl, combine the topping ingredients and blend with your fingers until crumbly. Set aside.

CAKE: In a small saucepan, combine the raspberries and 2 tablespoons orange juice over medium heat. Cook 5 to 10 minutes. Meanwhile, blend the remaining 2 tablespoons orange juice and cornstarch. Stir in the sugar if using. Add this combination to the saucepan. Continue cooking until thickened, about 5 minutes. Set aside.

   In a small bowl, mix together the cheese and sour cream until smooth. Set aside.

   Preheat the oven to 350 degrees and lightly oil a 9-by-13-inch baking pan. In a large bowl, stir together the flour, sugar, baking powder, baking soda, and salt. Make a well in the center. Pour in the melted butter, egg substitute, vanilla, and buttermilk. Stir until just moistened. Pour into the prepared pan.

Gently spread the cheese mixture on top within one inch of the edges. Top with the raspberry mixture. Sprinkle the topping over all. Bake until a toothpick inserted near the center comes out clean, about 45 minutes. Let cool. Cut in half lengthwise, then crosswise to make sixteen pieces.

PER SERVING: 238 calories; 7g protein; 39g carbohydrates; 6g fat (23 percent calories from fat); 2g fiber; 15mg cholesterol; 316mg sodium.

▪ PMS SOOTHERS ▪

Among the favorite PMS-craved foods is chocolate. And why not? The sweet-creamy nature of chocolate can prompt the manufacture of serotonin as well as the endorphins. The endorphins are your body's own stash of morphine, helping to alleviate pain and fostering general well-being. Other important PMS-soothers are vitamin B_6, and the minerals calcium and magnesium. The very worst food to eat: animal fats. Research indicates that the more animal fats you eat, the greater your likelihood of PMSing to the max.

HIGH-CALCIUM FOODS

Milk
Yogurt
Cheese
Green leafy vegetables
Broccoli
Enriched tofu
Enriched soymilk
Enriched orange juice
Enriched apple juice
Okra
Blackstrap molasses
Figs
Citrus fruits
Legumes

Cantaloupe-Peach Smoothie

Refreshing is the word that sums up this fruity concoction. It's a quick beta-carotene– and calcium-rich breakfast for busy mornings.

2 cups frozen sliced peaches
1 cup frozen cantaloupe chunks
½ cup nonfat plain yogurt

1 tablespoon soy protein powder
  or nonfat dry milk powder
  (optional)
2 tablespoons wheat germ
  (optional)

SERVES 2

Combine all the ingredients except the wheat germ in a blender and puree until smooth. (You may need to occasionally stop the blender to push down the frozen fruit with a wooden spoon.) Pour into two large glasses and sprinkle with the wheat germ, if using. Serve at once.

PER SERVING: 133 calories; 5g protein; 30g carbohydrates; 1g fat (7 percent calories from fat); 3g fiber; 1mg cholesterol; 51mg sodium.

Strawberry Sunrise Smoothie

Pretty and delicious, this smoothie is good for you too, with plenty of calcium and vitamin C.

2 cups frozen chopped
  strawberries
1 cup frozen sliced peaches
1 cup nonfat plain yogurt

½ to ¾ cup calcium-fortified
  orange-juice concentrate
Whole, fresh strawberries and
  mint leaves for garnish

MAKES 4

In a blender or food processor, puree the frozen strawberries, ⅔ cup of the yogurt, and about ½ cup orange-juice concentrate. Transfer to a bowl and place in the freezer.

Rinse the blender or food processor. Puree the peaches and remaining ingredients except the garnish.

In dessert glasses or bowls, layer the fruit mixtures, starting and ending with the strawberry blend. With a knife, swirl the smoothies to create an arc of peach. Garnish with the whole strawberries and mint. Serve at once.

PER SERVING: 165 calories; 4g protein; 37g carbohydrates; 0g fat (0 percent calories from fat); 3g fiber; 1mg cholesterol; 58mg sodium.

No-Knead Batter Bread

When you don't have the time or inclination to make bread from scratch, choose this tasty loaf. It's nearly fat-free, so try to resist the temptation to smear butter all over it. If you must have something on it, think marmalade.

1 cup whole-wheat flour
1½ cups unbleached white flour
¼ cup toasted wheat germ
¼ cup crushed bran cereal
3 tablespoons nonfat dry milk
½ teaspoon ground ginger

1 package active dry yeast
1½ tablespoons virgin olive oil
1⅓ cups water
3 tablespoons honey
⅔ teaspoon salt

SERVES 12

In a large bowl, mix together the whole-wheat flour, ½ cup unbleached white flour, wheat germ, cereal, dry milk, ginger, and yeast. Dribble the oil onto the mixture and stir. Set aside. In a small saucepan, heat the water, honey, and salt until hot to the touch, about 120 to 130 degrees. Pour slowly into the bowl, stirring constantly. With an electric mixer, beat at high speed for 3 minutes. Stir in the remaining 1 cup unbleached white flour.

Cover the bowl with plastic wrap and set in a warm place (about 80 degrees) for 10 minutes. Transfer the batter to a lightly oiled 5-by-9-inch loaf pan or 8-inch round cake pan. Cover loosely with a clean dish towel and let rise in a warm place until nearly doubled, about 30 minutes.

Bake until lightly browned and a toothpick inserted near the center comes out clean, about 40 minutes. Let cool slightly. Remove from the pan and cool thoroughly on a rack. Store in the refrigerator.

> PER SERVING: 141 calories; 5g protein; 25g carbohydrates; 2g fat (14 percent calories from fat); 2g fiber; 1mg cholesterol; 130mg sodium.

Orzo Spinach-and-Cheese Salad

Orzo is a tiny treasure of a pasta. Here it shows off a mixture of cheese, spinach, olives, and other taste treats.

½ pound uncooked orzo pasta
⅓ cup diced Asiago cheese or
   other favorite cheese (optional)
4 cups washed, trimmed, and
   torn spinach, lightly steamed
¼ cup chopped Kalamata olives

½ cup diced celery
¼ cup diced red onion
1 tablespoon virgin olive oil
2 tablespoons balsamic vinegar
Salt and freshly ground black
   pepper to taste

SERVES 4

Prepare the orzo according to the package directions. Rinse with cool water and drain. Stir in the cheese if using, spinach, olives, celery, and red onion. Combine the oil and vinegar, and drizzle over the salad. Toss lightly. Season with the salt and pepper. Chill. Serve cool or at room temperature.

> PER SERVING: 258 calories; 9g protein; 37g carbohydrates; 8g fat (28 percent calories from fat); 4g fiber; 9mg cholesterol; 181mg sodium.

Seven-Vegetable Casserole

This is great comfort food: Beaver Cleaver's favorite vegetables, topped with a mashed potato crust.

¼ cup red wine or Basic Vegetable Stock (page 247)

1 onion, sliced

2 teaspoons minced fresh garlic

1 cup thickly sliced white button mushrooms or other favorite mushrooms

1 celery stalk, sliced

¼ cup chopped red or green bell pepper

1 cup water

¼ to ½ cup low-sodium soy sauce or tamari

1 cup fresh or frozen corn kernels

1 cup fresh or frozen green peas or green beans

1 cup fresh or frozen sliced carrots

½ teaspoon dried oregano

¼ teaspoon dried thyme

Dash ground ginger

2 tablespoons cornstarch dissolved in ¼ cup water

1½ cups seasoned mashed potatoes

½ cup reduced-fat sharp cheddar cheese (optional)

MAKES 4

In a large saucepan, heat the wine or stock over medium heat and add the onion, garlic, and mushrooms. Simmer until the liquid is almost evaporated, about 10 minutes. Add the celery and bell pepper, and cook, stirring constantly, for 3 minutes more.

Add the remaining ingredients except for the dissolved cornstarch, mashed

HIGH-SELENIUM FOODS
Wheat bran
Rice bran
Broccoli
Cabbage
Celery
Cucumbers
Egg yolk
Fresh garlic
Milk
Cheese
Yogurt
Mushrooms
Onions
Wheat germ
Whole-grain flour

potatoes, and cheese if using, and simmer until the vegetable are barely tender, about 15 minutes. Stir in the dissolved cornstarch. Cook until thickened, about 3 minutes. Transfer the vegetable mixture to a lightly oiled 2-quart casserole dish.

Preheat the oven to 350 degrees. Spread the mashed potatoes evenly over the vegetable mixture. Sprinkle on the cheese if using. Bake until the top is lightly browned and the cheese is melted, about 25 to 30 minutes.

PER SERVING: 240 calories; 8g protein; 43g carbohydrates; 4g fat (14 percent calories from fat); 7g fiber; 2mg cholesterol; 901mg sodium.

Risotto Primavera

Risotto is Italy's finest contribution to rice cooking. Arborio rice is stirred and simmered until it's creamy but still has a "bite." Very simple to make, this dish spotlights the flavor of the vegetable you choose to add.

2 tablespoons butter or virgin olive oil
1 onion, diced
1 cup sautéed asparagus, eggplant, broccoli, mushrooms, or other favorite vegetable
8 cups Basic Vegetable Stock (page 247)

1 tablespoon saffron threads
2 cups uncooked Arborio rice
½ cup dry white wine
1 cup freshly grated Parmesan cheese
Salt and freshly ground black pepper to taste

SERVES 8

Melt the butter or heat the oil over low heat in a large, heavy-bottomed saucepan. Add the onion and one-half of the sautéed vegetables. Cook until the onion is translucent, about 10 minutes. Meanwhile, in another saucepan, simmer the stock over medium heat. Combine 1 cup of the warmed stock with the saffron and let stand.

Stir the rice into the onion-vegetable mixture and increase the heat to medium, stirring frequently, and cook until the rice appears chalky, about 5 minutes. Add the wine and stir until absorbed. Add the saffron mixture and then the stock, 1 cup at a time, stirring frequently. Add the remaining sautéed vegetables and continue cooking until the rice is creamy and tender but still has a bite. Gently stir in the Parmesan and season with the salt and pepper. Serve warm.

> PER SERVING: 270 calories; 9g protein; 41g carbohydrates; 7g fat (22 percent calories from fat); 3g fiber; 16mg cholesterol; 230mg sodium.

Chard Phyllo Pie

The phyllo (also spelled *filo*) makes a lovely crust for this calcium-rich pie. You may substitute spinach or kale for the chard.

¼ cup Basic Vegetable Stock (page 247)
¼ cup minced shallots
½ cup chopped white button mushrooms or other favorite mushrooms
1 teaspoon minced fresh garlic
1 tablespoon chopped fresh tarragon (or 1 teaspoon dried)
6 cups lightly steamed chard, well-drained

2 cups nonfat or part-skim ricotta cheese
1 egg, beaten
1 tablespoon fresh lemon juice
½ teaspoon ground nutmeg
Salt and freshly ground black pepper
Butter-flavored cooking spray
4 sheets phyllo
1½ tablespoons melted butter

SERVES 6

In a small skillet, heat the vegetable stock, shallots, mushrooms, garlic, and tarragon over medium heat. Cook, stirring occasionally, until the liquid evaporates, about 10 minutes. Set aside. In

a medium bowl, mix to-
gether the chard, ricotta,
egg, juice, nutmeg, and salt
and pepper. Set aside.

Preheat the oven to 350
degrees. Lightly spray an
8-inch square baking pan
with butter-flavored cooking spray. Using a pastry
brush and working speedily
because phyllo dries out
quickly, very lightly brush
the melted butter over each
phyllo sheet and stack them

> **HIGH-MAGNESIUM FOODS**
>
> Leafy green vegetables
> Almonds
> Cashews
> Soybeans
> Seeds
> Dairy products
> Avocados
> Apples
> Apricots
> Figs
> Peaches
> Beets
> Whole grains

on top of one another. Place the phyllo in the baking pan. Spoon
the chard mixture onto half of the phyllo, leaving a one-half-inch
edge. Gently lift the unfilled half of the phyllo over the chard,
tucking the edges under to seal. Lightly spray the top of the pie
with the butter-flavored cooking spray. Bake until golden brown,
about 45 minutes. Let cool slightly before cutting.

> PER SERVING: 161 calories; 17g protein; 15g carbohydrates; 4g fat
> (23 percent calories from fat); 1g fiber; 48mg cholesterol; 276mg so-
> dium.

Savory Potato Blintzes

Top on my list of dinner favorites are blintzes. My mom used to
serve them when I was a girl, and I'm still in love with them.

CREPES:

1 egg
¾ cup reduced-fat soymilk or
   skim milk

½ cup unbleached white flour
Dash salt

FILLING:

1½ cups Sour Cream 'n' Chive
     Whipped Potatoes (page 313)

GARNISH:

2 teaspoons butter   Chopped fresh chives
1 onion, sliced

Makes 8; serves 4

CREPES: Combine the crepe ingredients in a blender or food processor and whirl until smooth. Transfer to a bowl. Let stand 30
minutes. To cook, lightly oil an 8-inch nonstick skillet. Heat over
medium heat. Pour 2 or 3 tablespoons of the batter into the center
of the skillet, tilting it gently so the batter spreads to the edges. Cook
30 to 40 seconds. Loosen an edge of the crepe with a spatula and
flip over. Cook 15 seconds more. Slide the crepe onto a sheet of
waxed paper. Repeat this procedure until all of the batter is used
up, stacking the crepes between sheets of waxed paper.

FILLING: Place 3 tablespoons of the whipped potatoes in the center
of each crepe. Roll up, folding in the ends as you roll, to make
rectangular "packages." Place the blintzes in a lightly oiled baking
pan. Bake until golden, about 30 minutes.

GARNISH: Meanwhile, in a small skillet, melt the butter over medium heat and sauté the onion until very limp, about 15 minutes.
Set aside. Transfer the baked blintzes to a serving platter. Top with
the onions and chives. Serve warm.

PER SERVING: 183 calories; 6g protein; 32g carbohydrates; 4g fat (19
percent calories from fat); 3g fiber; 60mg cholesterol; 394mg sodium.

Sour Cream 'n' Chive Whipped Potatoes

Butter and milk weigh down the usual mashed potatoes. These are lightened by sour cream and flavored with chives.

8 potatoes, peeled and cut into chunks
Water to cover
2 tablespoons nonfat sour cream

2 tablespoons reduced-fat margarine
Salt to taste
1 to 2 tablespoons minced fresh chives

SERVES 4

In a large pot, bring the potatoes and water to a gentle boil over medium-high heat. Cook until fork-tender, about 20 minutes. Drain. Return the potatoes to the pot and add the sour cream and margarine. Whip with an electric beater until smooth. Season with the salt and garnish with the chives. Serve at once.

PER SERVING: 271 calories; 5g protein; 55g carbohydrates; 5g fat (16 percent calories from fat); 5g fiber; 5mg cholesterol; 64mg sodium.

Chocolate-Banana-Almond Pudding

When you're feeling out of sorts, this endorphin-boosting comfort food comes to the rescue. Choose a tofu that's fortified with calcium salts.

2½ cups mashed bananas
⅔ cup reduced-fat firm silken tofu
½ teaspoon almond extract
2 tablespoons cocoa powder, preferably Dutch process

¼ cup maple syrup
2 tablespoons toasted almond slivers for garnish

SERVES 6

Place all the ingredients except the almonds in a blender and process until smooth. Spoon into six dessert glasses. Chill for at least 1 hour. Garnish with the almond slivers. Serve cold.

PER SERVING: 156 calories; 4g protein; 33g carbohydrates; 2g fat (12 percent calories from fat); 3g fiber; 0mg cholesterol; 35mg sodium.

Chocolate Mousse with Berry Sauce

Light and fluffy, this mousse has just enough fat to perk up your endorphins but not so much that you feel weighed down. If the berries are sour, sweeten them with a tablespoon of honey or frozen juice concentrate before blending.

1 cup nonfat plain yogurt
⅓ cup semisweet chocolate chips
2 tablespoons prepared coffee
4 egg whites
¼ cup granulated sugar

½ pound frozen chopped
  strawberries or other berries
6 chocolate curls
Several sliced fresh strawberries
  for garnish

MAKES 6

Line a sieve with several layers of cheesecloth, spoon in yogurt, and allow to drain over a bowl in the refrigerator overnight. Bring to room temperature when you're ready to make the mousse.

Melt the chocolate in a double boiler, stirring frequently, or in a microwave on high at 30-second intervals. Combine with the yogurt and coffee in a metal bowl. Let cool to room temperature. In another metal bowl, beat the egg whites and sugar until soft peaks form. Very gently fold the egg mixture into the chocolate mixture, until just combined. Chill. Puree the strawberries in a blender. Pour into a bowl.

To serve, spoon 2 tablespoons of strawberry sauce on a small plate. Top with a scoop of mousse. Garnish with a chocolate curl and a few strawberry slices. Repeat with the remaining sauce, mousse, and garnishes. Serve at once.

PER SERVING: 131 calories; 1g protein; 20g carbohydrates; 3g fat (21 percent calories from fat); 1g fiber; 1mg cholesterol; 66mg sodium.

Chocolate Cupcakes

These cupcakes contain neither eggs nor dairy products, but no one will know. They're deliciously tender and chocolatey. If you must have frosting, make a thick glaze of Confectioners' sugar, unsweetened cocoa powder, and a little soymilk or dairy milk and spread it over the cupcakes.

1½ cups unbleached white flour
1 cup whole-wheat flour
1½ cups granulated sugar
½ cup unsweetened cocoa powder
1½ teaspoons baking powder
1 teaspoon baking soda

½ teaspoon salt
2 cups water
6 tablespoons safflower or canola oil
2 tablespoons white distilled vinegar
Confectioners' sugar

MAKES 24

Preheat the oven to 350 degrees. Lightly oil two 12-cup cupcake tins. (Do not use cupcake liners; the cake will stick to them.)

In a large bowl combine the flours, sugar, cocoa powder, baking powder, baking soda, and salt. In another bowl, mix together the water, oil, and vinegar. Pour into the dry ingredients and mix until just combined. Spoon the batter into the prepared pans and bake until a toothpick inserted into the center of a cupcake comes out clean, about 15 minutes.

Let cool. To remove, slide a knife around the perimeter of

each cupcake. Lightly sprinkle the cupcakes with Confectioners' sugar.

> PER CUPCAKE: 128 calories; 2g protein; 23g carbohydrates; 4g fat (27 percent calories from fat); 1g fiber; 0mg cholesterol; 128mg sodium.

Cherry Dump Cake

This not-too-sweet, simple dessert seems a cross between a cake and a muffin. It serves up a hefty dose of B vitamins.

½ cup whole-wheat flour
½ cup unbleached white flour
2 teaspoons baking powder
Dash ground nutmeg
¼ cup honey
¼ cup apple butter, preferably unsweetened

⅔ cup reduced-fat soymilk or skim milk
2 tablespoons butter, melted
One 16-ounce can sour cherries, unsweetened, with juice reserved
⅓ cup Confectioners' sugar

SERVES 8

Preheat the oven to 350 degrees. In a medium bowl, mix together the dry ingredients. Make a well in the center. Add the honey, apple butter, and milk. Stir until just moistened. Pour the melted butter into a lightly oiled, 8-inch round cake pan. Add the batter, and top with the cherries. Bake until a toothpick inserted near the middle comes out clean, about 35 to 40 minutes. Let cool.

Whisk a couple of tablespoons of the reserved cherry juice into the sugar to make a smooth icing. Dribble over the cake. Cut into wedges.

> PER SERVING: 180 calories; 3g protein; 36g carbohydrates; 3g fat (15 percent calories from fat); 2g fiber; 8mg cholesterol; 162mg sodium.

Double Chocolate Choco-Chip Cookies

If you adore chocolate and the endorphin lift it can give, you may think these cookies are heaven-made. Don't let the prunes and wheat germ fool you; the rich chocolate flavor comes through loud and clear.

⅓ cup pureed prunes, preferably unsweetened (see tip, below)
¾ cup granulated sugar
1 egg
4 tablespoons melted butter (or safflower or canola oil)
½ teaspoon vanilla extract
1 cup unbleached white flour

½ cup whole-wheat flour
⅓ cup unsweetened cocoa powder
¼ cup toasted wheat germ
½ teaspoon baking soda
½ teaspoon salt
¾ to 1 cup semisweet chocolate chips

MAKES 36; SERVES 18

Preheat the oven to 375 degrees. In a large bowl, blend the pureed prunes, sugar, egg, butter or oil, and vanilla extract. In another bowl, combine the flours, cocoa powder, wheat germ, baking soda, and salt. Add the dry ingredients to the wet ingredients, stirring until well blended. Stir in the chocolate chips.

Drop by teaspoonfuls onto baking sheets. Bake until the bottoms are lightly browned, about 8 minutes. Let cool slightly then remove to waxed paper. Store in an airtight container.

A Tip: If you don't have the time to puree your own prunes, buy prune butter, preferably unsweetened, or pureed prune baby food.

PER SERVING: 148 calories; 3g protein; 22g carbohydrates; 5g fat (30 percent calories from fat); 2g fiber; 19mg cholesterol; 126mg sodium.

Frozen Banana-and-Blueberry Parfaits

One of the best attributes of bananas, besides their high-potassium content, is that they mimic ice cream when frozen.

4 bananas, peeled and frozen overnight

1 cup frozen blueberries or sliced strawberries

1 tablespoon honey or granulated sugar (optional)

¼ cup nonfat plain yogurt or whipped cream (optional)

Blueberries for garnish

SERVES 4

Just before serving, cut the bananas into chunks and puree until smooth in a blender or food processor. Mix the berries and honey or sugar, if using. Spoon half of the banana puree into each of four parfait glasses or glass dessert bowls. Cover with the berries, then the remaining banana puree. Dollop the yogurt or whipped cream on top if using. Garnish with a few blueberries. Serve at once.

PER SERVING: 125 calories; 1g protein; 32g carbohydrates; 1g fat (7 percent calories from fat); 4g fiber; 0mg cholesterol; 3mg sodium.

▪ BODY BUILDERS ▪

To pump up your body, you need a mix of carbos and protein, with extra protein as needed for the demands of your sport, and ample antioxidants, especially the vitamins beta-carotene, C, and E, and the mineral selenium. Getting your fair share of the mineral boron is body-smart too. Some research suggests that eating foods rich in boron may raise testosterone levels in men and women, aiding muscle building. So which foods are boron biggies? Among the best are soy foods, including soymilk and tofu, and prunes, raisins, peanuts, and hazelnuts.

Nachos Bonitos

Nachos sold in fast-food joints are often an awful combination of oily chips and psychedelic-colored cheese. Here baked tortilla chips get a healthy fill of black beans, tomatoes, reduced-fat cheese, and other flavorful ingredients. Serve it as an appetizer, lunch, or part of dinner.

6 cups baked tortilla chips
½ to 1 cup grated reduced-fat cheddar or Monterey Jack cheese
½ cup nonfat sour cream
One 4-ounce can mild green chilies
1 teaspoon minced fresh garlic
1 teaspoon chili powder
½ teaspoon ground cumin
One 15-ounce can black beans, rinsed and drained
4 plum tomatoes, seeded and diced
¼ cup chopped scallions (green and white parts)
½ avocado, diced (optional)

SERVES 6

Preheat the broiler. Place the tortilla chips in a single layer in a baking pan. In a small bowl, combine the cheese, sour cream, chilies, garlic, and spices. Spread over the chips, completely covering them. Sprinkle the black beans, tomatoes, and scallions on top.

HIGH-MANGANESE FOODS

Apples
Apricots
Leafy green vegetables
Whole grains
Beets
Nuts

Broil until the cheese melts, about 3 minutes. Transfer to a serving platter. Sprinkle the avocado on top if using. Serve warm.

PER SERVING: 175 calories; 10g protein; 32g carbohydrates; 3g fat (15 percent calories from fat); 7g fiber; 8mg cholesterol; 338mg sodium.

Black Bean and Barley Soup

I've been a fan of barley ever since my introduction to it in Campbell's soup. I like it even better homemade, with legumes, carrots, onions, and seasonings.

2 cups uncooked black beans
Water for soaking
8 cups water
1 cup uncooked barley
2 onions, chopped
2 teaspoons minced fresh garlic
1 bay leaf
1 teaspoon dried oregano,
    crumbled
¼ teaspoon dried leaf thyme,
    crumbled

⅛ teaspoon cayenne pepper
3 medium carrots, pared and
    finely chopped
⅓ cup chopped fresh cilantro or
    fresh parsley
1 tablespoon red wine vinegar, or
    to taste
Sprigs of fresh cilantro and sour
    cream for garnish (optional)

SERVES 8

Cover the beans with water in a large saucepan. Let stand 8 hours or overnight. (Or to quick-soak beans, bring them to a boil in water over high heat and cook 2 minutes. Remove from heat and let stand 1 hour.) Drain. Return the beans to the saucepan and add the 8 cups fresh water, barley, half of the onion, garlic, bay leaf, oregano, thyme, and cayenne pepper. Bring to a boil over medium-high heat, then lower the heat, cover, and simmer 1½ hours, stirring occasionally. Add the remaining onion and the carrot. Cover and simmer 1½ hours more, adding additional water if necessary.

Place 1 cup of the soup in a food processor or blender and puree. Return to the saucepan. Stir in the cilantro or parsley and vinegar. Remove the bay leaf before serving. Garnish with sprigs of cilantro and a dollop of sour cream if desired.

PER SERVING: 279 calories; 19g protein; 55g carbohydrates; 1g fat (4 percent calories from fat); 15g fiber; 0mg cholesterol; 14mg sodium.

Tuscan White Bean and Herb Sandwich

This is my favorite sandwich spread: creamy, flavorful, and filling.

One 15-ounce can cannellini
beans, rinsed and drained
1 to 2 tablespoons fresh lemon
juice
3 to 4 tablespoons soymilk or
Basic Vegetable Stock (page
247)
1 to 2 teaspoons low-sodium soy
sauce or tamari
½ cup chopped fresh parsley

¼ cup chopped fresh basil
10 whole-grain rolls, sliced in
half lengthwise
Dijon-style mustard to taste
1 cucumber, sliced thinly
2 tablespoons chopped Kalamata
olives (optional)
Freshly ground black pepper to
taste

SERVES 10

Place the beans in a bowl and mash with a fork. Stir in the lemon juice, soymilk or vegetable stock, soy sauce or tamari, parsley, and basil. Combine thoroughly. Let chill for at least 30 minutes.

Preheat oven to 300 degrees. Heat the rolls until lightly toasted, about 10 minutes. Remove them from the oven and cover with a dish towel to keep warm.

Spread a thin layer of mustard on both halves of a roll. Spread ¼ cup of the bean mixture on the bottom half. Arrange several cucumber slices and olive pieces, if using, on top. Sprinkle with the pepper. Repeat this procedure with the remaining rolls, mustard, bean mixture, cucumber, olives, and pepper. Serve at once.

A Tip: Feeding a smaller crowd? Just use as many rolls as you need and refrigerate the remaining bean mixture. It keeps for several days.

PER SERVING: 161 calories; 8g protein; 28g carbohydrates; 2g fat (12 percent calories from fat); 7g fiber; 0mg cholesterol; 224mg sodium.

Grilled Felafel Pocket

A popular street food in the Middle East, felafel is the original "veggie burger." Customarily fried, this update is grilled indoors or out and adorned with the traditional yogurt-based sauce. Use the peanut butter option only if you cannot get your hands on a jar of tahini.

PATTIES:

1 teaspoon sesame oil or virgin olive oil
1 small onion, chopped
Two 15-ounce cans chickpeas, drained and rinsed
1 medium potato, boiled and peeled
¼ cup chopped fresh parsley

1 teaspoon minced fresh garlic
2 teaspoons ground cumin
2 teaspoons paprika
1 teaspoon salt
1 tablespoon tahini (sesame paste) or peanut butter
1 tablespoon fresh lemon juice

SAUCE:

1½ cups nonfat plain yogurt
2 tablespoons fresh lemon juice
1 tablespoon tahini or peanut butter
1 teaspoon minced fresh garlic
2 teaspoons ground cumin

3 tablespoons minced fresh parsley
4 pita rounds, warmed
2 cups thinly sliced romaine lettuce
8 thin tomato slices
Cayenne pepper sauce to taste

SERVES 4

PATTIES: In a small skillet, heat the oil over medium-high heat, swirling the pan to coat the bottom. Sauté the onion until soft, about 5 minutes. Transfer to a large mixing bowl. In a blender or food processor, puree the chickpeas and potato, and add to the mixing bowl. Add the remaining filling ingredients and combine thoroughly.

Preheat the broiler. Shape the mixture into eight patties. Place them on a lightly oiled baking sheet and broil until browned, about

5 minutes. Flip and broil the other side. Remove from the broiler. (Or place the patties on a barbecue grill to cook.)

SAUCE: Thoroughly combine the yogurt, lemon juice, tahini or peanut butter, garlic, cumin, and parsley. Set aside.

Cut each pita round in half, making eight pockets. Stuff each with a felafel pattie, lettuce, and tomato. Spoon the sauce on top and add a drop or two of cayenne pepper sauce. Serve warm.

> PER SERVING: 267 calories; 13g protein; 44g carbohydrates; 4g fat (14 percent calories from fat); 6g fiber; 1mg cholesterol; 209mg sodium.

Peapod-Mushroom Sauté and Cheese Wrap

A thick tortilla is a great base for this vitamin-bursting sandwich.

2 teaspoons virgin olive oil
½ onion, slivered
2 carrots, cut into matchsticks
8 white button mushrooms, sliced thickly
¼ cup diced red bell pepper
¼ cup dry red wine
1½ cups peapods, fresh or frozen

1 tablespoon low-sodium soy sauce, or to taste
2 tablespoons chopped fresh cilantro
Four 8-inch tortillas (see tip, below)
4 slices reduced-fat Swiss cheese

SERVES 4

In a skillet, heat the oil over medium heat and sauté the onion, carrots, mushrooms, and red bell pepper until softened, about 7 minutes. Add the red wine and peapods and cook 5 minutes more. Season with the soy sauce and cilantro. Set aside.

Heat the tortillas on a dry griddle over medium heat for 30 seconds, top with the cheese, and let melt, about 2 to 3 minutes. Place one-quarter of the sauté on each tortilla and fold over. Fasten with toothpicks. Transfer to individual plates. Serve warm.

A Tip: The best tortillas for this dish are the thicker, Mexican-style variety found in Hispanic markets and well-stocked super-markets.

PER SERVING: 272 calories; 6g protein; 30g carbohydrates; 8g fat (26 percent calories from fat); 4g fiber; 20mg cholesterol; 348mg sodium.

Mom's Best Spaghetti

The very first dish I learned to cook was spaghetti with a rich tomato-and-meat sauce. My mother's recipe wasn't a recipe per se, for it was never written down. While improvisation was welcome, it always included a can of tomato soup, ground beef, and Italian sausage in addition to the usual ingredients. This make-over retains a "meaty" flavor, but it fares far better on the nutrition scoreboard.

2 teaspoons virgin olive oil
1 onion, quartered and sliced
    crosswise
2 teaspoons minced fresh garlic
½ cup sliced white button
    mushrooms
1 green bell pepper, cored and
    sliced into strips
One 16-ounce can diced
    tomatoes with juice (or 3 ripe,
    flavorful tomatoes, chopped)
One 6-ounce can tomato paste
    mixed with ½ cup Basic
    Vegetable Stock (page 247) or
    water

Splash of dry red wine
Pinch of ground nutmeg
1 tablespoon chopped fresh
    oregano (or 1 teaspoon dried)
Salt and freshly ground black
    pepper to taste
1 cup frozen texturized vegetable
    protein (see tip, below)
4 vegetarian breakfast-style
    sausages, cut into chunks
    (optional)
¾ pound uncooked spaghetti

SERVES 8

In a large saucepan, heat the oil over medium-high heat, swirling to coat the bottom. Stir in the onion, garlic, and mushrooms, and sauté until the onion softens, about 5 minutes. Stir in the bell pepper and sauté 5 minutes more. Reduce the heat to medium. Add the diced tomatoes and tomato paste-and-broth mixture, stirring well. Season with the red wine, nutmeg, oregano, and salt and black pepper. Add the texturized vegetable protein and sausages if using.

Reduce the heat to medium-low and let simmer for at least 30 minutes. Meanwhile, bring a large pot of water to boil. Cook the spaghetti until al dente. Drain.

> ## THE NEW FAT MATH
>
> To figure the ideal number of fat grams for you, use these guidelines:
>
> Let's say you eat about 2,000 total calories a day, the amount for a typical, healthy adult woman. Assuming the fat percentage of 20 to 25 percent in the Ultimate version of my Power-Up Food Plan, you get to eat 44 to 56 fat grams.
>
> Other examples:
>
> 1,500 total calories, 33 to 42 fat grams daily.
>
> 2,500 total calories, 56 to 69 fat grams daily.
>
> 3,000 total calories, 67 to 83 fat grams daily.
>
> Knowing your day's worth of fat grams helps you choose the right foods, the ones that'll power up your mind, mood, and body. For instance, if you're shopping for soup on your way home from work, reading the "Nutrition Facts" may prompt you to pick lentil soup, with two grams of total fat and no saturated fat in a one-cup serving, over cream of mushroom soup, with seven grams of total fat, of which two and a half are saturated, in a one-cup serving.

Serve the spaghetti on a platter or individual plates, topped with a generous amount of the sauce. Serve hot.

A Tip: Look for frozen texturized vegetable protein, which is already seasoned, in well-stocked supermarkets and natural food stores. If you're unable to find it, substitute ½ cup dried texturized vegetable protein.

PER SERVING: 300 calories; 23g protein; 47g carbohydrates; 2g fat (7 percent calories from fat); 8g fiber; 0mg cholesterol; 221mg sodium.

Grilled Vegetable Kebabs with Pecan Wild Rice

Want to impress somebody? This dish is absolutely lovely and satisfying. If you think the tofu may not go over well with your guests, use portobello mushroom caps instead. When cooked, they smell and taste a lot like beef tenderloin.

WILD RICE:

3 cups Basic Vegetable Stock
(page 247)
1 cup uncooked brown rice

½ cup uncooked wild rice
½ cup chopped pecans, toasted

MARINADE:

¼ cup fresh lemon juice
¼ cup balsamic vinegar
2 tablespoons virgin olive oil

1 tablespoon minced fresh garlic
1 scallion (green and white
parts), minced

KEBABS:

¾ pound firm seasoned tofu, cut
into 36 one-inch cubes (see
tip, opposite page)
12 crimini mushrooms or white
button mushrooms
1 red bell pepper, cut into 12
one-inch chunks

1 onion, cut into quarters
1 zucchini, cut into 12
one-inch chunks
Fresh rosemary branches
(optional)

SERVES 6

WILD RICE: In a large saucepan, bring the stock to a boil, stir in the rices, cover, and lower the heat to medium-low. Cook until the liquid is absorbed, about 40 minutes. Sprinkle the pecans on top and toss gently.

MARINADE: Combine the ingredients and pour into a shallow dish. Set aside.

KEBABS: Alternately thread the tofu and vegetables onto six metal or bamboo skewers. Place in the marinade and let stand for at least 30 minutes. At outside cooking time, scatter the rosemary branches over the hot coals of your grill. (Or heat your broiler.) Place the kebabs on the grill or in the broiler. Grill, turning occasionally, until the vegetables are tender, about 5 minutes. Serve on top of the rice.

A Tip: You can find different kinds of seasoned tofu in well-stocked supermarkets and natural food stores. In a pinch, use plain firm silken tofu.

PER SERVING: 267 calories; 9g protein; 40g carbohydrates; 9g fat (27 percent calories from fat); 5g fiber; 0mg cholesterol; 33mg sodium.

Cheese Tortellini with Spinach Pesto and Roasted Red Pepper Sauce

With its red and green sauces, this dish is just right for Christmastime or any special occasion. It's particularly rich in antioxidants and calcium.

SPINACH PESTO:

1 cup frozen chopped spinach, thawed and squeezed dry
½ cup freshly grated Parmesan cheese
½ cup chopped fresh parsley
1 tablespoon minced fresh garlic
½ tablespoon virgin olive oil
½ teaspoon salt
Freshly ground black pepper to taste
Basic Vegetable Stock (page, 247), as needed

ROASTED RED PEPPER SAUCE:

3 red peppers, roasted (see tip, below)
½ tablespoon virgin olive oil
2 tablespoons balsamic vinegar
1 tablespoon minced fresh garlic
½ teaspoon salt

TORTELLINI:

3 cups cooked cheese tortellini
¼ cup very finely shredded
   Parmesan cheese (optional)

Chopped fresh parsley for
   garnish

MAKES 6

SPINACH PESTO: Place all the ingredients except the vegetable stock in a blender or food processor. Blend until very smooth, adding the stock as needed. Set aside.

ROASTED RED PEPPER SAUCE: Place all the ingredients in a blender or food processor and blend until very smooth. Set aside.

On four individual plates, pour some of the pesto on one half and some of the red pepper sauce on the other half. Top with the tortellini, sprinkle with the Parmesan, and garnish with the parsley.

HIGH-POTASSIUM FOODS
Orange juice
Bananas
Dried fruits
Bran
Peanut butter
Legumes

A Tip: To roast a bell pepper, hold it with tongs over a gas burner until blackened. Place in a paper bag, close, and let steam 10 minutes. Remove the charred skin with a paper towel.

PER SERVING: 246 calories; 12g protein; 30g carbohydrates; 8g fat (30 percent calories from fat); 3g fiber; 25mg cholesterol; 652mg sodium.

Three-Bean "Meaty" Chili

Serve this hot-as-you-like-it chili over thick, Mexican-style tortillas or whole-wheat couscous. Garnish with orange wedges and kiwifruit slices.

1 tablespoon virgin olive oil
1 onion, sliced
1 green or red bell pepper, seeded and diced
1 tablespoon chili powder
1 teaspoon ground cumin
6 white button mushrooms, chopped
¼ cup dry red wine, beer, or Basic Vegetable Stock (page 247)
1½ cups cooked kidney beans
1½ cups cooked black beans
¾ cup cooked white beans or chickpeas
One 28-ounce can crushed tomatoes

1 cup Basic Vegetable Stock or water
1½ cups texturized vegetable protein
½ teaspoon ground cinnamon
Salt and freshly ground pepper to taste
½ teaspoon cayenne pepper, or to taste
Additional splash of dry red wine (optional)
¾ cup reduced-fat cheddar cheese
½ cup nonfat sour cream
¼ cup chopped fresh cilantro for garnish

SERVES 6

In a large saucepan, heat the olive oil over medium-high heat, swirling the pan to coat the bottom. Sauté the onion, bell pepper, chili powder, and cumin until the onion is almost transparent, about 5 minutes. Add the mushrooms, cover, and cook 5 minutes more, stirring occasionally. Add the ¼ cup wine, beer, or stock; beans; tomatoes; 1 cup stock or water; and texturized vegetable protein. Reduce the heat to medium-low and let simmer at least 30 minutes.

Season with the remaining spices and additional wine if using.

Pour into individual bowls and top with cheese, sour cream, and cilantro. Serve warm.

PER SERVING: 371 calories; 29g protein; 52g carbohydrates; 6g fat (14 percent calories from fat); 15g fiber; 11mg cholesterol; 460mg sodium.

Lentil Ragout

A ragout is simply a thick sauce—a wonderfully seasoned sauce in this case. Enjoy it as is, but I prefer to spoon it over brown rice or couscous, or to stuff it into soft taco shells along with lettuce, tomato, and cucumbers.

3 cups water
1 cup uncooked lentils
1 teaspoon virgin olive oil
1 tablespoon minced fresh garlic
1 tablespoon chili powder
1 teaspoon ground cumin
2 scallions (green and white parts), sliced

1 green bell pepper, cored and diced
½ cup shredded carrot
One 6-ounce can tomato paste
1 tablespoon molasses, preferably blackstrap
1 tablespoon red wine vinegar
¼ cup chopped fresh cilantro for garnish

SERVES 6

In a medium saucepan, bring the water to a boil over medium-high heat. Add the lentils, return to a boil, cover, and reduce the heat to low. Let simmer until the lentils are tender but not mushy, about 25 minutes.

In a medium skillet, heat the oil over medium-high heat, swirling the pan to coat the bottom. Add the garlic, spices, and scallions, and sauté 3 minutes. Add the bell pepper and carrot and sauté 5 minutes more. Reduce the heat to medium and stir in the remaining ingredients except for the cilantro. Simmer 1 minute. Add to the cooked lentils, combining gently. Garnish with the cilantro.

PER SERVING: 167 calories; 10g protein; 30g carbohydrates; 2g fat (11 percent calories from fat); 10g fiber; 0mg cholesterol; 84mg sodium.

Moroccan Couscous with Chickpeas

The national dish of Morocco, quick-cooking couscous fluffs up like rice. Here it's spiced and paired with another Moroccan favorite: chickpeas.

2 teaspoons virgin olive oil
1 onion, thinly sliced
1 potato, boiled and diced
1 cup diced tomatoes
½ cup shredded carrots
½ teaspoon ground cumin
½ teaspoon turmeric
¼ teaspoon ground cinnamon
One 15-ounce can chickpeas, rinsed and drained

2 cups uncooked couscous
3 cups Basic Vegetable Stock (page 247)
¼ cup chopped fresh cilantro
Salt and freshly ground black pepper to taste
Cayenne pepper sauce to taste (optional)

SERVES 4

In a large saucepan, heat the oil over medium-high heat, swirling the pan to coat the bottom. Sauté the onion until softened, about 5 minutes. Reduce the heat to medium. Stir in the potato, tomatoes, carrots, and spices, and cook another minute, adding a tablespoon or two of water if necessary. Add the chickpeas, couscous, vegetable stock, and cilantro. Bring to a boil, cover, remove from the heat and let sit until the liquid is absorbed, about 5 minutes.

Fluff the couscous with a fork. Season with the salt, black pepper, and cayenne pepper sauce if using. Serve warm.

PER SERVING: 500 calories; 18g protein; 96g carbohydrates; 5g fat (9 percent calories from fat); 10g fiber; 0mg cholesterol; 31mg sodium.

■ IMMUNITY BOOSTERS ■

Strengthen your immunity by power-eating with a focus on foods particularly rich in antioxidants. Antioxidants scavenge extra free radicals that can wreak havoc with your body and cause disease. The best known antioxidants are beta-carotene, the precursor to vitamin A, vitamins C and E, and the mineral selenium. Along with eating good foods all the time, avoid those that can promote free radical production in the body, namely animal foods.

Tomato Soup with Garlic Croutons

Besides vitamin C, this meal starter has a good share of lycopene, a phytochemical believed to stave off illness.

2 teaspoons canola or safflower oil
1 onion, thinly sliced
2 stalks celery, trimmed and thinly sliced
2 teaspoons minced fresh garlic
4 cups seeded and diced tomatoes (either perfectly ripe and flavorful or canned)
3 tablespoons chopped fresh basil (or 1 tablespoon dried)
2 cups warmed Basic Vegetable Stock (page 247)

1 tablespoon brown sugar (if needed to reduce acidity)
½ to 1 teaspoon salt
Freshly ground black pepper to taste
4 slices medium-textured bread, cut into 1-inch cubes
Olive oil cooking spray
1 cut garlic clove
Chopped fresh parsley for garnish

SERVES 6

In a large soup pot, heat the oil over medium-high heat. Sauté the onion, celery, and garlic until the onion is transparent, about 5 minutes. Reduce the heat to medium. Add the diced tomatoes, basil, and stock, and cook for 10 minutes. Add the sugar if using, salt, and pepper.

Meanwhile, preheat the oven to 350 degrees. Place the bread cubes in a single layer on a baking sheet, spray lightly with olive oil cooking spray, and toast until crisp, about 2 to 4 minutes. Rub the croutons with the garlic clove.

Divide the soup among six bowls and garnish with the croutons and parsley. Serve at once.

PER SERVING: 92 calories; 3g protein; 16g carbohydrates; 3g fat (29 percent calories from fat); 3g fiber; 0mg cholesterol; 244mg sodium.

Vidalia Onion Soup

Vidalias are superb sweet onions that caramelize beautifully. Another is Washington State's Walla Wallas. All onions are rich in phytochemicals and may have important health benefits. In this soup, you get a whole onion in a serving—and no bad breath.

2 tablespoons canola or safflower oil
6 Vidalia or Walla Walla onions, thinly sliced (see tips, below)
1 tablespoon balsamic vinegar
1 to 2 tablespoons dry red wine
Pinch of granulated sugar
8 cups Basic Vegetable Stock (page 247)

1 to 2 tablespoons miso (see tips, below)
Salt to taste
6 slices French bread or sourdough bread
6 tablespoons freshly grated Parmesan cheese

SERVES 6

In a large soup pot, heat the oil over medium-high heat. Stir in the onions, coating them with the oil. Reduce the heat to medium-low and cook, stirring frequently, until the onions are limp, about 40 minutes. Add the vinegar, wine, and sugar, and continue stirring as the onions caramelize, about 15 minutes more.

Pour in the stock. Bring the soup to a boil over medium-high heat, reduce to medium-low, and let simmer for 30 minutes. Season with the miso and salt. Divide the soup among six oven-proof bowls.

Heat the broiler. Place a slice of bread in each bowl, pushing it down to soak it. Sprinkle each with 1 tablespoon Parmesan. Place the bowls in a broiler, 2 or 3 at a time, until the cheese melts, about 2 minutes. Serve at once.

10 SUPER-QUICK DINNERS

When you need a meal on the table now, quickly survey your pantry and fridge, and make one of these. Fill out your meal with fresh fruit and a salad or steamed vegetables.

1. Grilled or sautéed vegetables in teriyaki sauce, served in tortilla wraps
2. Cheese ravioli with your favorite tomato sauce
3. Store-bought veggie burgers on buns with all the trimmings
4. Burritos or quesadillas made with refried beans, cheese, tomatoes, scallions and lettuce, and topped with salsa
5. Bagels or English muffins, split and topped with tomato sauce, mozzarella cheese and vegetables of your choice, then broiled
6. Leftover or store-bought soup with hunks of crusty bread
7. Whole-grain pancakes or waffles with berries
8. Leftover brown rice mixed with a can of vegetarian baked beans and garnished with minced scallion
9. A main-dish salad of lettuce, a variety of vegetables, legumes, dried fruit and nuts
10. Phone your favorite takeout restaurant and put a rush on your order

A Few Tips:

No Vidalias or Walla Wallas in sight? Choose Spanish onions, which are large, yellow, and, most important, mild.

Miso is a flavorful, salty paste made from fermented soybeans. It adds depth to soup and other dishes. The darker the miso, the stronger the flavor. Look for miso in natural food stores.

PER SERVING: 263 calories; 8g protein; 41g carbohydrates; 8g fat (26 percent calories from fat); 7g fiber; 4mg cholesterol; 360mg sodium.

Russian Borscht

During a trip to Moscow to adopt my daughter Julia, we stayed at my friend Ludmilla's cozy apartment and she served us traditional country fare, including borscht and hearty bread. My version of her lovely soup is chunkier, but just as tasty. If you like beets, you'll clamor for second helpings.

3 medium beets
1 teaspoon virgin olive oil
1 onion, sliced
1 carrot, diced
2 quarts Basic Vegetable Stock (page 247)
2 potatoes, peeled and cut into chunks
½ head cabbage, cut into 1-inch-square pieces

One 14½-ounce can diced tomatoes, drained
Salt and freshly ground black pepper to taste
1 tablespoon minced fresh garlic
1 tablespoon finely chopped fresh dill
¼ cup nonfat sour cream

SERVES 8

Preheat the oven to 300 degrees. Place the beets in a small baking pan, and bake until tender, about 40 minutes. Let cool, then peel and shred coarsely. Set aside.

In a medium skillet, heat the oil over medium heat and cook the onion and carrot for 15 minutes. Meanwhile, in a large soup pot, bring the stock to a boil over medium-high heat, add the potatoes and cabbage, and cook 15 minutes. Add the tomatoes, beets, and sautéed vegetables. Season with the salt and pepper. Cook until heated through, about 10 minutes. Remove from the heat. Add the garlic and dill to the soup. Cover and let stand 10 minutes.

At serving time, pass the small bowl of sour cream to garnish.

PER SERVING: 85 calories; 3g protein; 18g carbohydrates; 1g fat (11 percent calories from fat); 4g fat; 1mg cholesterol; 140mg sodium.

Creamy Broccoli Soup

Back by popular demand, this recipe debuted in my book *The Vegetarian Child*. It gets raves from kids and adults alike, at least those who appreciate one of the healthiest vegetables on Earth.

2 cups chopped fresh broccoli, ½ cup set aside
3½ cups Basic Vegetable Stock (page 247), ½ cup set aside
4 potatoes, peeled and cubed

½ onion, chopped
½ to 1 tablespoon chopped fresh cilantro
Salt and freshly ground black pepper to taste

SERVES 6

In a large soup pot, bring all the ingredients—except the set-aside broccoli and stock and the salt and pepper—to a boil over medium-high heat. Cover, reduce the heat to medium, and cook until tender, about 20 minutes.

Puree the soup, a batch at a time, in a blender or food processor. Be sure to fill the blender or food processor no more than two-thirds full. Return the pureed soup to the pot. Add the remaining stock, season with the salt and pepper, and simmer 5 minutes.

Pour the soup into six individual bowls and garnish with the reserved broccoli. Serve warm.

PER SERVING: 92 calories; 3g protein; 21g carbohydrates; 1g fat (10 percent calories from fat); 3g fiber; 0mg cholesterol; 12mg sodium.

The Best Spinach Salad

Even spinach "haters" go back for seconds of this antioxidant-packed salad.

8 cups loosely packed, trimmed
  and torn spinach
½ cup dry sherry
2 tablespoons fresh lemon juice
¾ cup dried apricots, diced

1½ tablespoons virgin olive oil
¼ teaspoon salt
Generous sprinkling of freshly
  ground black pepper
2 tablespoons chopped pecans

SERVES 8

Place the spinach in a large serving bowl. In a small saucepan, mix together the sherry, lemon juice, and apricots and heat to a simmer. Cover and remove from heat. Let stand 20 minutes. Stir in the oil, salt, and pepper. Pour the dressing over the spinach and toss well. Sprinkle the pecans on top.

PER SERVING: 87 calories; 2g protein; 10g carbohydrates; 4g fat (40 percent calories from fat); 3g fiber; 0mg cholesterol; 113mg sodium.

Simple Green Salad

Did you know that romaine lettuce boasts a delightful share of vitamins and minerals, while the too-common iceberg has next to none?

SALAD:

1 small head romaine lettuce,
  torn into bite-sized pieces
1 small head red leaf lettuce, torn
  into bite-sized pieces
2 scallions (white part only), cut
  lengthwise into thin strips

3 carrots, grated
1 cucumber, halved lengthwise,
  seeded, and chopped

DRESSING:

2 tablespoons balsamic vinegar
1 tablespoon virgin olive oil
¼ teaspoon salt

Sprinkling of freshly ground
  black pepper

SERVES 8

SALAD: In a large serving bowl, combine the salad ingredients.

DRESSING: In a small bowl, whisk together the vinegar, oil, salt, and pepper. Pour over the salad and toss.

Smart Note: This salad is perfect for dressing up with favorite add-ons. Some possibilities are chopped marinated artichoke hearts, sun-dried tomatoes, zucchini rounds, roasted red bell pepper strips, chopped red onion, toasted sunflower seeds, toasted pine nuts, chopped dried fruit, crumbled feta, chopped Asiago cheese, and sprinklings of garden-fresh herbs.

> PER SERVING: 49 calories; 2g protein; 7g carbohydrates; 2g fat (37 percent calories from fat); 3g fiber; 0mg cholesterol; 88mg sodium.

Sweet Potato, Apple, and Pear Salad

This salad brings together the sweetness of vitamin-packed ingredients in a citrus dressing.

DRESSING:

¼ cup orange juice
3 tablespoons raspberry vinegar
   or other favorite vinegar
1 tablespoon virgin olive oil

1 teaspoon grated orange rind
   (see tip, opposite page)
½ teaspoon salt

SALAD:

1 baked sweet potato, peeled and
   cubed
1 Granny Smith apple, cored and
   sliced
1 Gala apple or other favorite
   red apple, cored and sliced
1 pear, cored and sliced

¼ cup chopped shallots
2 cups watercress, stemmed
2 cups Bibb lettuce, gently torn
   into bite-sized pieces
2 tablespoons toasted chopped
   pecans

SERVES 6

DRESSING: Whisk together the dressing ingredients. Set aside.

SALAD: In a medium bowl, combine the potato, apples, pear and shallots, and toss with half of the dressing. Line a serving platter with the watercress. Arrange the potato, apples, pear, shallots, and Bibb lettuce on top. Pour the remainder of the dressing on top. Garnish with the pecans.

A Tip: Use an organic orange. Oranges with bright color have been dyed. The dye is not meant for eating.

> PER SERVING: 115 calories; 2g protein; 20g carbohydrates; 4g fat (32 percent calories from fat); 3g fiber; 0mg cholesterol; 186mg sodium.

Cinnamon Baby Carrots with Pecans

This naturally sweet side dish teems with beta-carotene and vitamin E.

1 pound baby carrots	1 tablespoon ground cinnamon
¾ cup dry white wine or Basic Vegetable Stock (page 247)	Dash ground nutmeg
	Salt to taste
2 tablespoons apple juice concentrate	2 tablespoons pecans

SERVES 6

In a saucepan fitted with a cover, cook the carrots in the wine or stock and the apple juice concentrate over medium heat, stirring occasionally until the liquid evaporates and the carrots are barely fork-tender, about 15 minutes. Sprinkle with the cinnamon, nutmeg, and salt. Stir to coat. Cook 1 or 2 minutes more. Garnish with the pecans.

> PER SERVING: 68 calories; 1g protein; 8g carbohydrates; 2g fat (25 percent calories from fat); 3g fiber; 0mg cholesterol; 29mg sodium.

Greens Sauté with Fennel

With a Mediterranean flavor, this side dish is simply superb—and high in beta-carotene and vitamins C and E.

1 red bell pepper, cored and
    thinly sliced
1 tablespoon minced fresh garlic
½ cup water
6 cups washed, trimmed, and
    torn chard

2 tablespoons minced feathery
    part of a fennel bulb
2 to 4 tablespoons prepared
    pesto
¼ to ½ cup nonfat plain yogurt
    (optional)

SERVES 6

In a large skillet over medium heat, cook the red bell pepper and garlic in the water until the pepper is soft, about 5 minutes. Stir in the chard, then cover and cook until the leaves are tender, about 2 minutes. Add the fennel, pesto, and yogurt if using and stir until well-combined.

> PER SERVING: 31 calories; 1g protein; 3g carbohydrates; 2g fat (58 percent calories from fat); 1g fiber; 1mg cholesterol; 104mg sodium.

Quick Spinach Rice Pilaf

This dish can be a light entree or a substantial lunch when served with soup and sliced fruit. It's teeming with beta-carotene, B vitamins, and iron.

1 tablespoon red wine
1 cup chopped white button
  mushrooms
2 cups cooked brown rice
One 10-ounce package frozen
  chopped spinach, thawed
1 teaspoon low-sodium soy
  sauce, or to taste

1 teaspoon vegetable bouillon
  powder
1 egg, lightly beaten
¼ cup reduced-fat cheddar
  cheese
1 tablespoon toasted wheat germ
⅔ cup tomato sauce (optional)

SERVES 4

In a saucepan, heat the wine over medium heat and cook the mushrooms until softened, about 5 minutes. Meanwhile, in a medium bowl, combine the other ingredients except for the wheat germ and tomato sauce. Add the mushrooms. Transfer to a 1-quart casserole dish. Sprinkle the wheat germ on top. Microwave on high for 5 minutes. Let stand 5 minutes more, then stir with a fork. Top with the tomato sauce if desired.

PER SERVING: 208 calories; 13g protein; 30g carbohydrates; 5g fat (22 percent calories from fat); 5g fiber; 63mg cholesterol; 263mg sodium.

Ratatouille

No cream sauces in this classic Provencal stew: only the freshest, most flavorful vegetables. Serve it over couscous, saffron rice, or another favorite grain.

1 medium eggplant
2 teaspoons virgin olive oil
2 zucchini, sliced thinly
Basic Vegetable Stock (page 247), as needed
1 onion, sliced
1 tablespoon minced fresh garlic
2 bell peppers (green, red, or yellow), cored and sliced
4 to 5 plum tomatoes, peeled (see tip, below) and chopped
1 tablespoon fresh chopped basil (or 1 teaspoon dried)
1 tablespoon fresh chopped oregano (or 1 teaspoon dried)
Salt and freshly ground black pepper to taste
Cayenne pepper to taste
Herb vinegar of choice (optional)

SERVES 4

Peel and cut the eggplant into one-inch cubes; let sit in a colander 30 minutes then pat dry. In a large skillet, heat the olive oil over medium-high heat, swirling to coat the bottom of the pan. Add the eggplant and zucchini and cook, stirring frequently, until the vegetables are golden, about 10 minutes. Pour in a few tablespoons of the stock if the skillet becomes dry. Set eggplant and zucchini aside.

Sauté the onion and garlic in the skillet for a few minutes. Add the bell peppers and cook until softened, about 5 minutes. Add the tomatoes, herbs, salt, pepper, and cayenne; reduce the heat to low, cover, and cook another 5 minutes. Stir in the reserved eggplant and zucchini and cook until everything is tender, about 20 minutes more. Serve warm or chilled with a splash of herb vinegar if using.

A Tip: To peel tomatoes, make two slits in the tops. In a pot of boiling water, immerse the tomatoes for 30 seconds and remove them with a slotted spoon. When cool enough to handle, slip off the skins, cut open, and remove the seeds.

PER SERVING: 105 calories; 4g protein; 19g carbohydrates; 3g fat (26 percent calories from fat); 6g fiber; 0mg cholesterol; 18mg sodium.

Baked Eggrolls with Sweet-Sour Sauce

The typical eggroll is fried and fat-heavy. These are baked and filled with some of the richest antioxidant vegetables.

FILLING:

1 tablespoon sesame oil

2 scallions (green and white parts), chopped

2 carrots, cut into thin matchsticks

6 dried shiitake mushrooms, soaked until soft in hot water and thinly sliced

½ cup julienned red bell pepper

2 tablespoons chopped fresh cilantro

½ to 1 teaspoon peeled and minced gingerroot

Dash cayenne pepper

1 tablespoon low-sodium soy sauce or tamari

1 cup cooked bean thread noodles

2 cups shredded bok choy

WRAPPERS:

16 eggroll wrappers

Sesame oil for brushing

SAUCE:

½ cup orange juice or pineapple juice

½ cup rice vinegar

¼ teaspoon garlic powder

2 teaspoons arrowroot dissolved in 1 tablespoon low-sodium soy sauce or tamari

MAKES 16; SERVES 4

FILLING: In a wok or large skillet, heat the oil over medium-high heat and sauté the scallions, carrots, mushrooms, and bell pepper for 3 minutes. Add the remaining filling ingredients. Sauté 3 minutes more. Remove from the heat.

WRAPPERS: Lay a wrapper on your work surface with a corner facing you. Place a scant ¼ cup of the vegetable mixture in a horizontal rectangle across the center of the wrapper. Fold the bottom corner over the vegetable mixture. Fold in the right and left corners. Then wet the top corner with a bit of water and roll up the eggroll tightly. Repeat with the remaining wrappers and filling.

Preheat the oven to 400 degrees. Place the eggrolls on baking sheets. Brush with the oil and bake until lightly browned, about 10 minutes.

SAUCE: In a saucepan, combine the juice, vinegar, and garlic powder over medium-high heat and let simmer. Pour in the dissolved arrowroot and cook until thickened, about 5 minutes. Serve with the eggrolls.

PER SERVING: 428 calories; 12g protein; 82g carbohydrates; 6g fat (12 percent calories from fat); 4g fiber; 10mg cholesterol; 676mg sodium.

Pacific Rim Coleslaw

With its beta-carotene and vitamins E and C, this picnic food is for anytime.

1 tablespoon sesame oil
¼ cup rice vinegar
½ teaspoon salt
1 head savoy cabbage, thinly sliced
1 cup shredded carrots

2 scallions (white and green parts), sliced
2 tablespoons lightly toasted sesame seeds

SERVES 8

In a large bowl, whisk together the oil, vinegar, and salt. Add the cabbage, carrots, and scallions and toss well. Sprinkle the seeds on top. Serve at once or cover and refrigerate.

PER SERVING: 47 calories; 1g protein; 5g carbohydrates; 3g fat (57 percent calories from fat); 2g fiber; 0mg cholesterol; 150mg sodium.

Three-Bean Salad with Honey-Mustard Dressing

Here's an American favorite redone, with a lot less fat.

DRESSING:

4 tablespoons red wine vinegar
1½ tablespoons virgin olive oil
4 teaspoons Dijon-style mustard

2 teaspoons honey
¾ teaspoon salt

SALAD:

2 cups green beans, steamed
One 15-ounce can wax beans,
    drained and rinsed
One 15-ounce can kidney beans,
    drained and rinsed

½ cup sliced red onion
1 cup chopped red bell pepper
½ cup chopped celery
½ cup chopped fresh parsley

SERVES 6

DRESSING: Whisk together the vinegar, oil, mustard, honey, and salt in a small bowl. Set aside.

SALAD: In a medium bowl, combine the green beans, wax beans, kidney beans, onion, bell pepper, celery, and parsley. Pour the dressing over it and toss to mix. Let stand, covered, at room temperature for 2 hours or refrigerate overnight.

PER SERVING: 163 calories; 7g protein; 26g carbohydrates; 4g fat (22 percent calories from fat); 8g fiber; 0mg cholesterol; 378mg sodium.

Chilled Strawberry Soup

Begin or end your meal with this vitamin C–delicious soup. Be sure to wash the strawberries well to remove any pesticide residues.

2 cups sliced fresh strawberries,   2 tablespoons honey
    chilled   1 to 1½ cups plain nonfat yogurt
3 tablespoons orange juice   4 cantaloupe shells (optional)

SERVES 4

In a blender or food processor, puree the first four ingredients, reserving ¼ cup strawberries. Pour into four chilled bowls or the cantaloupe shells. Garnish with the reserved strawberries.

> PER SERVING: 91 calories; 4g protein; 19g carbohydrates; 1g fat (10 percent calories from fat); 2g fiber; 1mg cholesterol; 45mg sodium.

■ MEMORY MANAGERS ■

As we age, our memory invariably wanes. You can slow this process by eating foods rich in B vitamins, especially thiamine, niacin, B_6, B_{12}, pantothenic acid, and folic acid, as well as the minerals zinc, magnesium, and manganese and the antioxidants beta-carotene and vitamins C and E. Most important, get your fill of choline, the precursor to the memory-manager neurotransmitter acetylcholine. Choline-rich foods include egg yolks, soy, wheat germ, whole wheat, peanuts, and pecans.

Raspberry-Peach Smoothie

Here's another quick breakfast drink. It delivers choline-containing soy, beta-carotene, vitamin C, calcium, potassium, and other health-promoting phytochemicals.

⅔ cup frozen unsweetened   1 banana, peeled and frozen
    raspberries   4 ounces reduced-fat soft silken tofu
1 peach, peeled, pitted, and   1½ cups calcium-fortified orange
    frozen   juice

MAKES 2

Combine all the ingredients in a blender or food processor and puree until smooth.

> PER SERVING: 233 calories; 6g protein; 49g carbohydrates; 2g fat (8 percent calories from fat); 7g fiber; 0mg cholesterol; 90mg sodium.

Spring Rolls with Peanut Dipping Sauce

As an appetizer or a side to an Asian dinner, these spring rolls encase a crunchy and antioxidant-packed filling. The addictive peanut sauce contains choline, so dip without guilt.

FILLING:

½ cup cooked vermicelli
2 tablespoons rice vinegar
1 scallion (green and white parts), chopped fine
2 carrots, shredded
½ cup water chestnuts, chopped fine

1 cup mung bean sprouts
½ cup shredded bok choy
⅓ cup chopped fresh cilantro
1 tablespoon chopped fresh mint
50 wonton wrappers

SAUCE:

1 cup canned unsweetened coconut milk (see tip, below) or Basic Vegetable Stock (page 247)
2 tablespoons minced onion
2 teaspoons peeled and grated gingerroot
1 teaspoon minced fresh garlic

¼ cup creamy peanut butter
1 tablespoon low-sodium soy sauce or tamari
1 tablespoon brown sugar
½ teaspoon curry powder (optional)
Cayenne pepper sauce to taste

MAKES 50; SERVES 10

FILLING: Cut the vermicelli into 2-inch strands. Place in a medium bowl and toss with the vinegar. Stir in the scallion, carrots, water chestnuts, bean sprouts, bok choy, and herbs. Dip a wonton wrapper in water. Place it on a dry surface with a corner pointing toward you and blot away excess moisture. Spread a heaping tablespoon of the filling in the center of the wrapper. Fold up the bottom edge of the wrapper over the filling, fold in the sides, and roll up tightly. Place on a platter lightly oiled with sesame oil. Repeat with the remaining filling and wrappers.

SAUCE: In a small saucepan, bring ⅓ cup of the coconut milk or stock to a boil over medium-high heat. Add the onion, ginger, and garlic. Reduce the heat to medium-low and simmer until the liquid has nearly evaporated, about 7 minutes. Stir in the peanut butter and slowly add the remaining milk or stock. Add the remaining ingredients. Simmer, stirring frequently, until the sauce is thickened, about 10 minutes.

A Tip: Coconut milk is sold in Asian markets and some well-stocked supermarkets.

> THE DIRTIEST DOZEN
>
> Think twice before pigging out on the foods on a list compiled by the Environmental Working Group after reviewing records of the U.S. Food and Drug Administration. These foods had the highest residue levels (before washing) of forty-two common produce items.
>
> On the plus side, experts say washing your produce in water removes 25 to 50 percent of chemical residues. Peeling some produce items, like cucumbers, and discarding the outer leaves of head lettuce and cabbage also reduces your exposure.
>
> Strawberries
> Green and red bell peppers
> Spinach
> Cherries
> Peaches
> Cantaloupe (Mexican)
> Celery
> Apples
> Apricots
> Green beans
> Grapes (Chilean)
> Cucumbers

PER SERVING: 207 calories; 7g protein; 32g carbohydrates; 6g fat (27 percent calories from fat); 2g fiber; 4mg cholesterol; 337mg sodium.

Skinny Egg Salad Sandwiches

Eating typical egg salad can turn your blood to sludge and set you on the path to heart disease. This version retains enough choline—remember, eggs are among its primary sources—to aid your brain but uses antioxidant-rich ingredients in place of some cholesterol, fat, and calories.

6 hard-boiled eggs, diced
2 celery stalks, trimmed and diced
½ red bell pepper, cored and diced
1 baked red potato, diced
⅔ cup plain nonfat yogurt
⅓ cup low-fat cottage cheese
1 tablespoon honey

½ teaspoon minced fresh garlic
¼ cup minced fresh parsley
   (optional)
Salt and white pepper to taste
1 small loaf French bread, cut
   into 16 ½-inch slices
1 tablespoon paprika

SERVES 8

In a large bowl, combine the eggs, celery, bell pepper, and potatoes. In a small bowl, whisk together the yogurt, cottage cheese, honey, garlic, and parsley. Pour the dressing over the egg mixture and gently combine. Season with the salt and pepper. Cover and refrigerate at least 30 minutes.

Spread about ⅓ cup of egg salad on a slice of bread. Sprinkle a little paprika on top and cover with another slice of bread. Do the same with the remaining egg salad and bread slices.

> PER SERVING: 242 calories; 12g protein; 35g carbohydrates; 6g fat (21 percent calories from fat); 2g fiber; 161mg cholesterol; 407mg sodium.

PB&J Updated

Who says PB&J is for kids only? First, it's delicious. Second, it's quick to make. Third, it's choline-rich.

2 tablespoons smooth or chunky
   peanut butter
2 tablespoons nonfat or part-
   skim ricotta cheese
½ tablespoon toasted wheat germ

4 slices whole-wheat bread
1 to 2 tablespoons of your
   favorite fruit spread or low-
   sugar preserves

In a small bowl, thoroughly blend the peanut butter and ricotta cheese. Spread half of the mixture on a slice of bread and sprinkle with half of the wheat germ. Top another slice of bread with half of the fruit spread or preserves, and make a sandwich. Repeat with the remaining peanut butter mixture, wheat germ, and preserves.

PER SERVING: 277 calories; 13g protein; 37g carbohydrates; 11g fat (36 percent calories from fat); 5g fiber; 1mg cholesterol; 393mg sodium.

Savory Vegetable Frittata

What's the difference between a frittata and an omelette? A frittata is peasant food while the oh-so-delicate omelette is, well, delicate. Both are flavorful, but I'd choose a frittata any day.

1 to 2 teaspoons virgin olive oil
¼ cup diced onion or scallions (green and white parts)
½ red or green bell pepper, diced
¼ cup sliced white button mushrooms or other favorite mushrooms
1 tablespoon fresh herbs, such as tarragon, basil, or oregano (or 1 teaspoon dried)

Basic Vegetable Stock (page 247), as needed
2 eggs or 1 cup egg substitute
¼ cup reduced-fat cheese of choice, such as cheddar, Swiss, or mozzarella, shredded
Salt and freshly ground black pepper to taste

SERVES 4

Preheat the oven to 350 degrees. Heat the oil over medium heat in a 10-inch oven-proof skillet. Add the onion or scallions, bell pepper, mushrooms, and herbs, and sauté until the vegetables are soft, about 10 minutes, adding a splash or two of vegetable stock to keep skillet from becoming dry.

Whisk the eggs or egg substitute and cheese in a medium bowl. Pour the mixture into the skillet, season with salt and pepper, and stir gently until it begins to set, about 3 minutes. Lift up an edge with a nonmetal spatula, tilt the skillet, and let the eggs run underneath. Let cook 20 seconds more, then lift another edge and repeat the process until the top is no longer runny but not completely set.

Place the skillet in the oven for a few minutes, checking frequently to avoid overcooking. An overcooked frittata gets a tad tough and less delicious than it could be. Cut into wedges and serve warm.

> PER SERVING: 120 calories; 13g protein; 4g carbohydrates; 6g fat (46 percent calories from fat); 1g fiber; 116mg cholesterol; 222mg sodium.

Cheesy Potato-Egg Casserole

This anytime dish has surprisingly little fat—only 8 grams a serving—and lots of serotonin-friendly carbos and choline-rich eggs. You may also serve it cold, cut into squares, as an appetizer.

2 teaspoons canola or safflower oil
4 potatoes, preferably Yukon Gold, peeled, quartered, and thinly sliced
2 eggs or ½ cup egg substitute
4 egg whites, beaten (optional)
2 cups low-fat small-curd cottage cheese
½ to 1 cup reduced-fat Monterey Jack or cheddar cheese

¼ cup freshly grated Romano or Parmesan cheese
¼ cup unbleached white flour
1 tablespoon chopped fresh tarragon (or 1 teaspoon dried)
1 teaspoon baking powder
½ teaspoon salt
3 tablespoons chopped pimentos

SERVES 8

In a large nonstick skillet, heat the oil over medium heat. Cook the potatoes until lightly browned, about 10 minutes. Remove from the heat.

Preheat the oven to 350 degrees. Lightly oil a 9-by-13-inch baking pan. In a large bowl, combine the remaining ingredients except the pimentos. Add the potatoes and stir. Pour into the prepared pan. Sprinkle the pimentos on top. Bake until golden, about 35 minutes. Serve warm.

> PER SERVING: 229 calories; 19g protein; 23g carbohydrates; 8g fat (30 percent calories from fat); 2g fiber; 78mg cholesterol; 618mg sodium.

Tandoori Kebabs

Tandoori is a barbecue à la Pakistan and other parts of Asia. The *tandoor,* or barrel-shaped oven, lends an intriguing smoky flavor mimicked by American-style grills. The preparation time requires a good two days, but the cooking is quick.

TOFU AND MARINADE:

One 10½-ounce package
   reduced-fat firm silken tofu
   or seasoned firm tofu,
   frozen then thawed
1 cup Basic Vegetable Stock
   (page 247)

¼ cup low-sodium soy sauce or
   tamari
1 scallion (green and white
   parts), sliced
2 teaspoons minced fresh garlic

2 tablespoons nutritional yeast
   (see tip, below)
1 tablespoon dried crumbled sage
1 teaspoon peeled and grated
   gingerroot
¼ teaspoon ground saffron
   (optional)

SAUCE KEBAB:

1 cup plain nonfat yogurt
2 tablespoons fresh lemon juice
1 onion, diced
2 teaspoons minced fresh garlic
1 teaspoon curry powder
1 teaspoon turmeric
½ teaspoon ground cumin
Dash ground cloves
Cayenne pepper sauce to taste

1 green bell pepper, cored and
   cut into 12 one-inch pieces
12 cherry tomatoes
12 white button mushrooms caps
6 bamboo skewers
6 chapatis or pita rounds
4 cups cooked basmati rice
6 lime wedges

Serves 6

TOFU AND MARINADE: Cut the tofu into about 18 one-inch cubes. In a shallow pan, mix together all the marinade ingredients. Gently transfer the tofu to the pan, cover, and let marinate in the refrigerator for at least 24 hours and up to 2 days, stirring occasionally.

SAUCE: Mix all the sauce ingredients in a medium bowl. Add the tofu cubes, covering them with the sauce completely. Cover and refrigerate overnight.

Heat a barbecue, indoor grill, or oven broiler. Thread each bamboo skewer with 2 bell pepper pieces, 2 tomatoes, 2 mushroom caps, and 3 tofu cubes, alternating them on the skewer. Grill or broil, basting with the sauce, until slightly charred on all sides, about 10 minutes.

Once cooked, place a skewer in a chapati or pita round. Remove the skewer. Serve with the rice, lime wedges, and any leftover sauce.

A Tip: Nutritional yeast has a nutty or cheesy flavor. You can find it in natural food stores and the supplement section of some large supermarkets.

PER SERVING: 385 calories; 16g protein; 78g carbohydrates; 2g fat (6 percent calories from fat); 5g fiber; 1mg cholesterol; 506mg sodium.

Peanutty Oat Cookies

Rich in choline, these lower-fat peanut butter cookies are memorable (please pardon the pun).

¼ cup pureed prunes, preferably unsweetened
½ cup granulated sugar
1 egg
3 tablespoons creamy peanut butter
½ teaspoon vanilla extract

¾ cup unbleached white flour
½ cup quick-cooking rolled oats
½ teaspoon baking soda
¼ teaspoon salt
¼ cup chopped peanuts

Makes 24; serves 12

Preheat the oven to 375 degrees. In a medium bowl, thoroughly combine the pureed prunes, sugar, egg, peanut butter, and vanilla. In another bowl, combine the flour, oats, baking soda, and salt. Stir the dry ingredients into the wet ingredients. Add the nuts, and stir until combined.

Drop the batter by spoonfuls onto oiled baking sheets. Bake for 8 minutes. Let cool on paper towels. Store in an airtight container.

PER SERVING: 122 calories; 4g protein; 18g carbohydrates; 4g fat (31 percent calories from fat); 1g fiber; 18mg cholesterol; 122mg sodium.

Soy-Good Strawberry Sherbet

This icy dessert makes eating soy foods and vitamin-rich fruit easy and fun—and you'd never, ever guess there was tofu in it.

1 cup chilled low-fat vanilla
soymilk
1 tablespoon honey
½ teaspoon vanilla extract

4 ounces reduced-fat soft or firm
silken tofu, chilled
2½ cups frozen chopped
strawberries

Serves 4

Combine all the ingredients except the strawberries in a blender or food processor and puree until smooth. Add the strawberries and puree again. Spoon into four dessert dishes and freeze 1 to 2 hours. Serve cold.

PER SERVING: 92 calories; 5g protein; 19g carbohydrates; 1g fat (10 percent calories from fat); 2g fiber; 0mg cholesterol; 53mg sodium.

With an emphasis on whole foods from cuisines around the world, the recipes in part 3 may have a few new-to-you ingredients. Here are definitions and information on the use of each. I've added in a few extras that do not appear in the recipes. You'll find them at natural foods stores, well-stocked supermarkets and ethnic markets.

Agar-agar: This flavorless sea vegetable sets mixtures just like gelatin. It's sold in three forms: powder, stick, and flakes.

Amaranth flour: This highly nutritious flour has a wonderfully distinctive flavor, so use it in small quantities when you add it to baked goods. If you can't find it, simply grind amaranth seeds.

Asafetida: This garlicky spice is used in Indian cooking.

Barley malt syrup: Made from sprouted barley, this dark, thick sweetener can replace honey or molasses in many baked goods. Its main sugar is maltose.

Brown rice syrup: Mild-flavored and expensive, this sweetener is made from cooked, fermented brown rice. It can replace honey in many baked goods.

Couscous: Technically a pasta, couscous (pronounced *kooz-kooz*) seems more like a grain. It absorbs water like other grains and can be fluffed with a fork. The refined variety is lighter and fluffier than whole-grain couscous.

Fructose: Though fructose appears naturally in fruit, the type sold in stores is even more refined than table sugar (sucrose). Nonetheless, fructose is helpful to diabetics, because it is more slowly digested. It's almost twice as sweet as table sugar, so you need less of it.

Granulated sugarcane juice: To make this sweetener, sugarcane juice is dehydrated and milled. It can replace sugar in recipes. Like other sweet-eners, except for iron-rich blackstrap molasses, it contains few nutrients.

Kudzu: Made from the root of this plant (pronounced *kood-zoo*), this white starchy substance can thicken puddings and sauces.

Millet: This mild grain makes a delicious side dish to spicy and savory entrees.

Miso: This thick, salty paste is made from cooked, aged soybeans. The lighter varieties of miso have milder flavors, the darker have stronger flavors. It's best known as a soup base.

Nutritional yeast: Packed with protein, iron, and some B vitamins, this nutty- and meaty-flavored yeast can be sprinkled on casseroles and soups. Use just a little (about ¼ teaspoon daily) at first, because it causes flatulence in some people. It's not meant for baking as is baker's yeast.

Quinoa: An ancient grain with a distinctive flavor, quinoa (pronounced *KEEN-wa*) is a delicious choice for pilafs. Rinse before cooking to remove any bitterness.

Seitan: This "meaty" food (pronounced *say-TAHN*) is actually the gluten protein of wheat. Its flavor varies with the herbs and spices it's cooked in.

Soba, udon: These Asian noodles are flavorful and protein-rich. Soba is made from buckwheat and wheat flours, and udon from wheat alone. Both somewhat resemble spaghetti noodles.

Tahini: This smooth, thick paste is similar to peanut butter but made from sesame seeds.

Tamari, shoyu: With a flavor almost identical to soy sauce, tamari and shoyu are used to season a variety of dishes. Tamari comes from wheat, and shoyu from soybeans and wheat.

Teff: This tiny grain with a faint chocolate flavor and a jellylike consistency when cooked hails from Africa, where it's used to make the flatbread *injera*. It works well in some baked goods.

Tempeh: Made from cultured soybeans, this food (pronounced *TEM-pay*) has a mild to pungent flavor, which becomes stronger with age.

Texturized vegetable protein: Also known by its acronym, TVP, this meat substitute is a dehydrated soy product fashioned from the flakes that remain after the extraction of oil from soy. It's sold as flakes, granules, and chunks, either plain or flavored. To use, reconstitute TVP in water and add it to saucy mixtures, like chili, spaghetti sauce, sloppy joes, and stews. It doesn't work well alone, as the primary ingredient in "meat" loaf, for instance.

Triticale: A hybrid of rye and wheat, this grain has extra protein and a hearty flavor.

Turbinado sugar: This sugar has not been bleached. It's devoid of nutrients except for calories.

Vegetarian Worcestershire sauce: With a zippy flavor just like regular Worcestershire sauce, this type has no anchovies.

APPETIZERS & SNACKS

SOUPS

ENTREES

SIDE DISHES

DESSERTS

BREAKFAST

SANDWICHES

BAKED GOODS

ET CETERA

Of Trees and Skinned Knees

High up in the tree I sat, hidden by the late spring leaves, every one of them new, perfect. This was my sanctuary—the place where I felt safe and secure, where I first encountered God, viscerally.

My eyes looked down at the ground, a muddy black-brown. I was a good twenty feet higher, unafraid, for the tree held me like a mother. Above I caught a glimpse of the heavens: Crayola-blue sky and white puffy clouds like in a child's drawing. A contemplative girl, I wondered what lay beyond the heavens I could see. Another place of beauty, of safety and security, like my tree, but better?

I, as do many others, see a synergy of mind (both brain and mood), body, and spirit. They are not separate, as Rene Descartes would have us believe. Mind, body, and spirit are interdependent: What you eat affects all of you, including your spiritual self, that part of you with the desire to know from which we came and to where we're headed. It is the essence of our souls.

The question of heaven dogged me for many seasons as we grew—the tree and me. Springtime was my favorite. Tiny buds let loose to shoots, green leaves, and even greener leaves. Watching growth in microcosm comforted me in a way I couldn't quite put a name on back then. Now I know it as hope, for as my tree came to life after a harsh winter, I sensed the spiritual lesson that I, too, would somehow, someway, make it up the hills and through the valleys of childhood. My tree was always there, waiting for me, to embrace me, to cover me with its love.

As shorter days signaled the coming autumn, its clothing turned an orangey red, and leaf by leaf it became naked. I hated the winter. My beloved sanctuary looked dead. It was bare, silent, alone. Who would warm it now?

Oh, yes, the snow. The snow would blanket it, lovelier than any seamstress could, and I saw finally, as I exchanged pigtails for prom dresses, the value in letting go. More spiritual lessons I learned: that beauty is only skin deep, that in being naked—vulnerable, really—I could reach deep into myself and know the true me, that after winter there was another spring, a glorious spring, when what appeared dead rustled, wiggled, and hopped to life.

This wasn't my first resurrection lesson. Back in the summer of 1968, when I was six years old and learning how to ride a two-wheeler, my knees knew only scabs. I could handle the straightaways just fine; the corners threw me—and I mean threw me. To the ground I would fall, a knee slamming into the sidewalk, a scab reopened. Another spiritual lesson: the power of healing, which came not from me—for all I did was wash and Band-Aid my hurts—but from something, Someone, greater than me. It was the same Someone I sensed in my tree lessons.

Though I lacked a formal spiritual upbringing, I nonetheless touched the power I now call God, or, more accurately, God touched me. (I use the pronoun *he* to describe God, though *she* also works, for the God I know incorporates maleness and femaleness. Our inept language cannot come close to capturing his/her essence.)

God taught me this truth: I am weak, like my skin, which tore so easily, while he is strong, the tree that towers in mightiness, beauty, and trustworthiness, with roots as expansive as its branches, anchoring it in the soil, from which it drinks up living water. Once I learned this seen/unseen lesson of the tree, I knew I could lean on it, on him, but not on me.

There was a time in which I played God. I believed I could do anything I set my mind to in my own power. I thought, *Why do I need God, when I can rely on me?* And so I worshiped the god of self-sufficiency and bought in to the popular universalist notion of our culture: that whatever you believe, whomever you embrace, as long as it works for you, it's fine—with you, with me, with everybody. This philosophy sounds really good. It's politically correct and seductive: tolerance with a capital *T*.

While I respect people whose spiritual views differ from mine—a number of whom are family—we all are created by the Creator, clay in the hands of the capable Potter. He loves me as much as he loves anyone else: a child molester, a mass murderer, a prostitute, a junkie. He cannot love any less or any more, for he is love.

My spiritual journey reminds me of a treasure map. The route is circuitous, through hollowed logs, into swamps and snakepits, up cliffs, across swinging bridges, into fields of flowers, onto mountaintops, into valleys, onto grassy plains. It is the narrow road the Bible speaks of. No one would choose it of their own accord. But when God taps your shoulder, as he did mine, inviting you to come, to experience spirit power, while he walks at your side, always, who could say no?

I am vaguely familiar with the teachings of many of the world's religions: Buddhism's Four Noble Truths, Islam's Koran, Hinduism's karma and reincarnation, and Judaism's adherence to the Law and Talmud. In each of these religions, the way to heaven, to increased spirituality, or to whatever's termed the ideal God state is through self.

For me, gentle nudges of the Spirit, the wind, a friend's hug, a child's bright eyes, the outstretched hand of a homeless person, the miraculous healing of a disease, the Bible and answered prayer—whether *yes, no,* or *wait*—are a few of the ways I experience the Living God, for he speaks to me through people, circumstances, his Word, and, yes, a tree.

The tree anchors me in the holy ground of my life.

It is grace.

It is pain.

It is victory.

It is spirit power.

If you have questions or comments, you may reach the author at this address:

Lucy Moll
c/o Perigee Books
375 Hudson Street
New York, New York 10014